TONY&TINA
COLOR
ENERGY

TONY&TINA

®

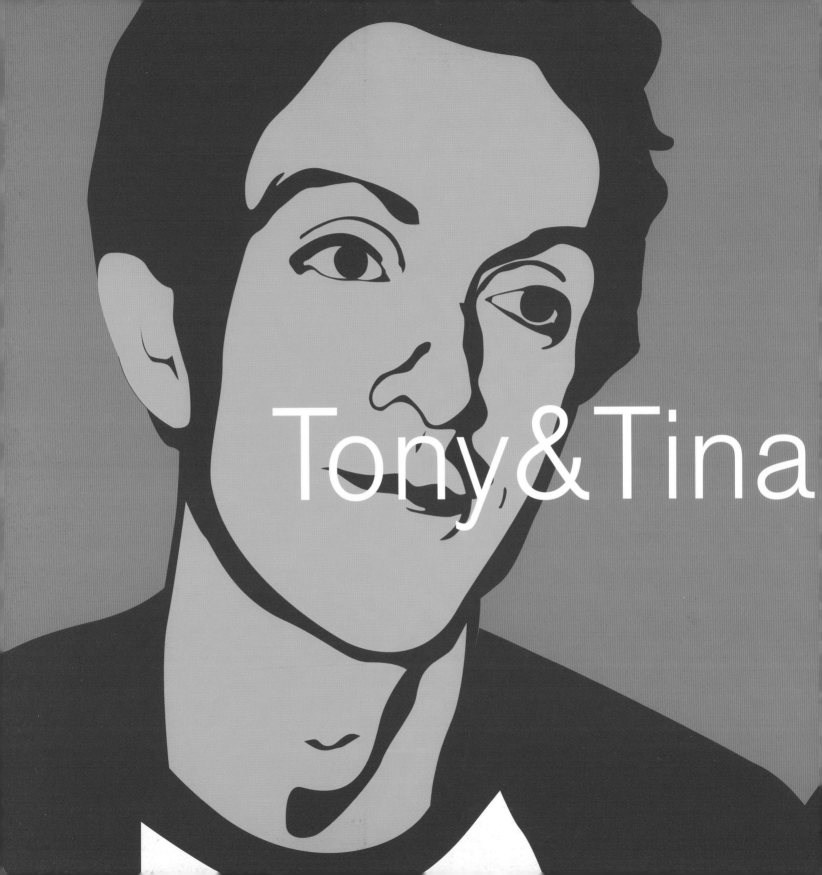

Tony&Tina

Color Energy

How Color Can Transform Your Life

Cristina Bornstein and Anthony Gill

Simon & Schuster · New York / London / Toronto / Sydney / Singapore

SIMON & SCHUSTER
Rockefeller Center
1230 Avenue of the Americas
New York, NY 10020

Photography and illustration credits appear on page 158.

Designed by MEMO Productions, New York
Manufactured in Italy
10 9 8 7 6 5 4 3 2 1
Library of Congress Cataloging-in-Publication Data is available.
ISBN 0-7432-1792-6

Tony&Tina Color Energy reflects the ideas and personal experiences of the
authors. It is not intended to be used as a guide for independent self-healing or
diagnosis. The authors make no medical claims regarding the effectiveness
of the exercises set forth within this book.

The I AM / The Divine Mind

In this lifetime, many minds are waking to the truth
That our reality is created by our thought.
Our understanding of the true nature of illness and disease is now
    in a quantum shift.
The fate of man is to become conscious creator.

The universal mind is all, regardless of the concepts we attach to it
Because we stand in the way of the light
We are the cause of the shadows in our life.

We will learn to let go of expectations
And walk into every moment with detached reverence
As observers with no judgments.
We will each watch the wondrous unfolding of our dreams.

The truth will be the prime focus of our humanity.
Love is all
Is the truth that sets us free.
    —Anthony Gill

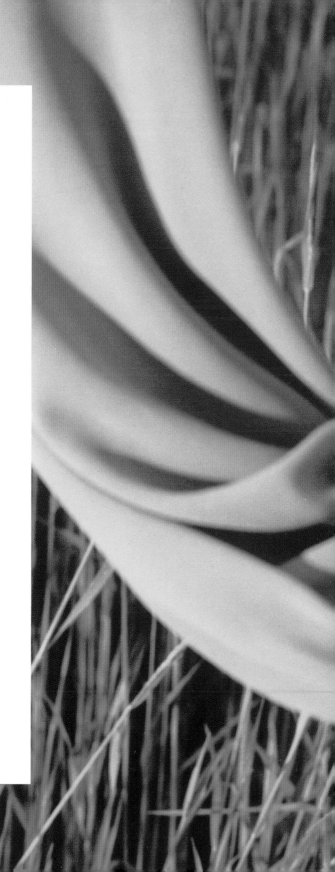

Contents

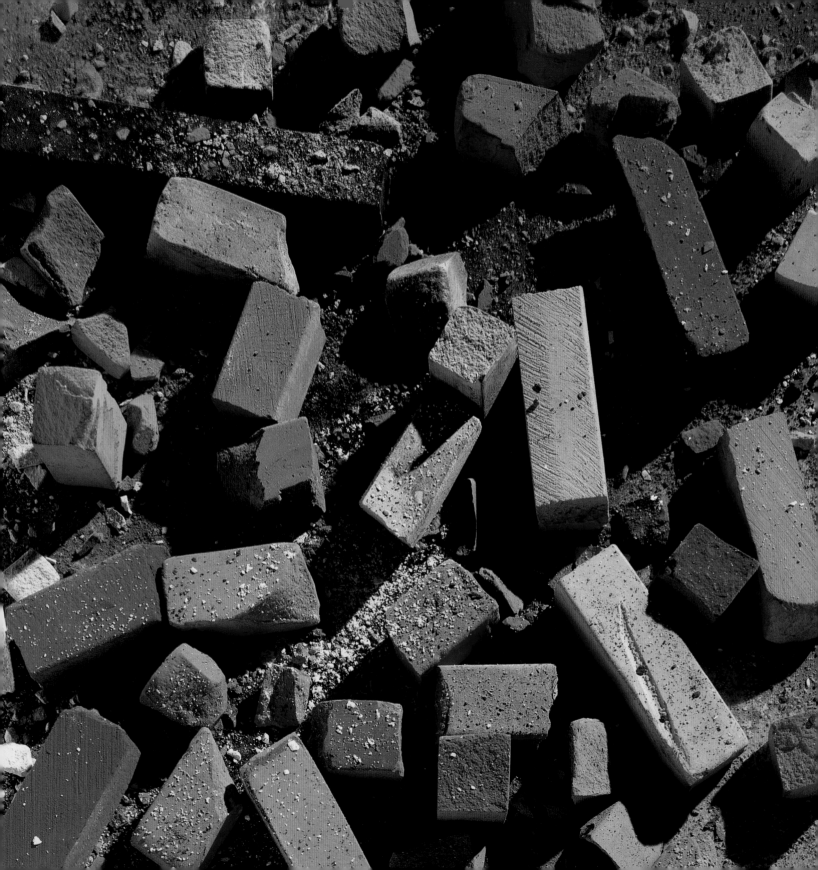

Introduction

 Tina: *When I was a teenager, I had a succession of blue dreams. For about a week straight, I dreamt I was surrounded by the most beautiful blue I've ever seen, even to this day. Nothing in particular ever happened in these dreams. I was just enveloped in blue and I would wake up feeling amazing, as if I had been fed huge amounts of love.*

At the time, I thought these dreams meant I was supposed to change my name to Blue. I desperately tried to get all my friends to call me that—only one did. Knowing what I do now, I have a better idea of what these dreams were about. I had a troubled childhood and blue is very healing for children. It eases loneliness and encourages individuality. My higher self was feeding me the healing color energy I needed and also teaching me that bathing in color energy is an effective way to find comfort and ease anxiety.

 Tony: *On Sunday afternoons, when I was a kid, my family would always watch the TV series* High Chaparral. *It became a sort of ritual. The character I identified with was named Blue. He was my inspiration, my alter ego. I would imagine that I was Blue and would have fantasies about going off and rescuing people and saving the world. I didn't know it then, but blue affects our capacity for self-expression, enabling us to speak out about what we believe. What better quality for a trainee superhero?*

When Cristina told me about her blue childhood dreams and I told her about pretending to be Blue, we could almost hear the strains of The Twilight Zone *theme swelling in the background.*

Every culture since the beginning of history has been aware of the power of color. It's been used to placate the gods, to ease passage into the next life, and to symbolize season, direction, rank, and royalty. Color has also long been recognized as a vital healing force. The Egyptians are thought to have built color therapy chambers in their pyramids; in fabled Atlantis, people were healed by color energy in a crystal dome; the Chinese still cure illness with foods and herbs of certain colors. In early cultures, jewelry set with precious gems was worn not merely for show but also to protect the wearer from harm and disease. Only since the advent of our "age of reason" have we forgotten the power and magic of color. Today we are coming full circle, back to the future. At this point in time, there is a growing awareness of the scientific truth behind the magic of color. That truth is energy.

Have you ever wondered why you always wear a certain color blue, or why you insist on using only green file folders, or why you had to throw out that chair just because it was orange? The answer is energy. Every color gives off its own particular vibration, and, like tuning forks, we respond to it. In a very real way, color influences our energy system and affects both our physical and emotional well-being. Consider our friend Karen: she comes home from work and almost always puts on a green sweatshirt. Green energy encourages feelings of love. While she may not be aware of green's therapeutic effects, Karen automatically envelops herself in this consoling color after a stressful day. All of us are unconsciously drawn to the color energy we need, and we literally feed our bodies with it.

Our intention in writing this book is to make the unconscious process of taking in color energy a conscious one. We'll explain how color works, how energy works, and show how you can introduce color into your life and positively influence your well-being on every level.

Albert Einstein taught that all material objects, including the physical body, consist of energy suspended in a timeless, flowing field. He showed that matter is actually composed of quanta, which in turn are made of invisible vibrations. In effect, that means our bodies are pure energy; we exist in a state of constant transformation. As Deepak Chopra explains: "This quantum field isn't separate from us—it *is* us. Although your senses report that you inhabit a solid body in time and space, this is only the most superficial layer of reality. Your body is something far more miraculous.... Every cell is a miniature terminal connected to the cosmic computer.... The unseen world is the real world and when we are ready to explore the unseen levels of our bodies, we can tap into the immense creative power that lies at our source."

Understanding the body as an ever-changing system of energy has gained wide acceptance in the twenty-first century thanks to the work of Chopra, Carolyn Myss, and many others. We are beginning to understand how our bodies, minds, and spirits are affected by the electromagnetic vibrations from within as well as from without. We have begun to accept that the vibrations of color, sound, aroma, thought, movement, flower essences, and gemstones can heal our bodies and our souls. We've learned that energy medicine—whether in the form of creative visualization, meditation, acupuncture, shiatsu, reiki healing, hands-on healing, rolfing, aromatherapy, feng shui, tai chi, chi gong, yoga, or color therapy—helps balance the frequencies of malfunctioning cells and restores us to our natural state of radiant well-being. Most of these practices are ancient. We are fortunate to live in a time where their therapeutic value can be understood and measured scientifically, a time when they are available to us to enhance our lives.

The global shift in consciousness about the nature of energy has resulted in a growing interest in alternative therapies. Prestigious hospitals such as Sloan-Kettering in New York City have opened alternative therapy centers and offer hands-on healing to postoperative patients. Spas offer shiatsu, sports centers acupuncture. Hospital rooms are painted in colors that encourage healing, and disturbed adolescents are placed in bubble-gum-pink rooms to calm them.

Countless books and articles on energy medicine tell us how to meditate, how to increase our energy, how to visualize ourselves rich, even how to raise our IQs by listening to Mozart. Vibrational remedies are now available in a variety of commercial forms. Instead of waking to a jarring buzz, we can rise to the scent of an aromatherapy alarm clock. When the pressures of urban living give us a headache we can be cured with a special machine that gives off blue light. We are really starting to understand that everything is quite literally energy (even money, which we already know as "cashflow" and "currency").

Some years earlier, in Trinidad, Tony had learned about the seven energy centers in the body from a Hindu teacher who used a different color of the spectrum to represent each one. At the time, the significance of the seven colors passed him by as so much esoteric blather. Even though he had studied the effects of color at art school, he didn't know what to do with the information until he met Cristina. Our mutual interest fueled our passion to explore the transformational effects of color. We ravenously devoured anything we could find on the subject of color therapy. We reveled in the idea that, by using the right colors, we might change self-destructive patterns, be healthier, and gain a higher level of consciousness.

The true nature of vibrational healing was revealed to us when we were at a particularly low point in our lives. We were artists but we weren't art stars. We were in and out of work. We felt that we had a compelling purpose in life, but the problem was, we weren't sure that being struggling artists was part of it. Then something crucial happened. We stumbled on a book called *Creative Visualization* by Shakti Gawain in which she explains that thought itself is energy and that our thoughts have a magnetic pull. We create our own reality by drawing to us the types of people and situations, positive and negative, that preoccupy us. Unless we understand this law of attraction ↓

and start visualizing the life we want, we create our reality by default, usually with disappointing results. Reading and rereading this book ignited something deep within us. Shakti's book gave voice to something we had dimly perceived but could never put into words, and suddenly we felt as though we were awakening from a coma. To realize we could consciously and positively create the reality we desired was an amazing and self-empowering discovery. By practicing the law of attraction, we became conscious creators. As we acknowledged and exercised our intuition more and more, we began to have the courage to live by doing what felt right. Meanwhile, we began to focus on color therapy.

As we slowly began to unlock our powers as visualizers, we continued to read, particularly the books by Carolyn Myss about her study of the energy centers and by Faber Birren, who has been researching the nature of color for decades. Ted Andrew's *How to Heal with Color* became our bible, as did *Wheels of Light,* an amazing book by Rosalyn Bruyere. Other books, listed in the bibliography, added to our understanding. As we progressed, we continued our spiritual practice, attending workshops and training sessions. The Tibetan initiation and empowerment sessions organized by the Nachung Foundation, founded by His Holiness, the Dalai Lama, were especially inspiring and deepened our understanding of the subtle energies of our actions and their consequences.

We decided to focus on practicing the principles of color therapy, and found ways of determining what colors we needed at any particular time. We adapted the color exercises we learned and practiced them on ourselves.

When a friend approached us to create a cosmetics line, we realized that this was the ideal high-profile platform from which to spread awareness of creative visualization, aroma, and color therapy. We wanted to play our part in contributing to an evolving global consciousness. Our intention was, and is, to share with as many people as possible the color therapy tools that can be used every day to create happiness, health, and greater abundance.

From our personal experience we know that color can positively affect the body's energy system. It is a vibrational remedy that can be used to heal and transform. Using the information in this book, you will learn how to use the power of color energy to positively affect your energy system and create the reality you truly desire.

Cristina Bornstein
Tony Gill

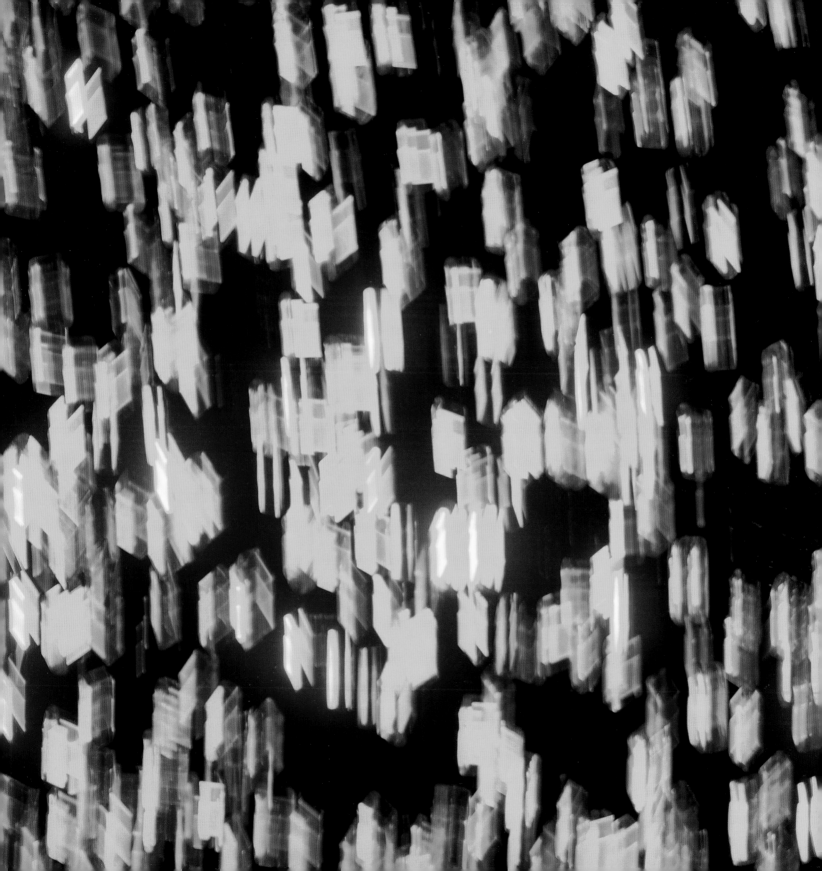

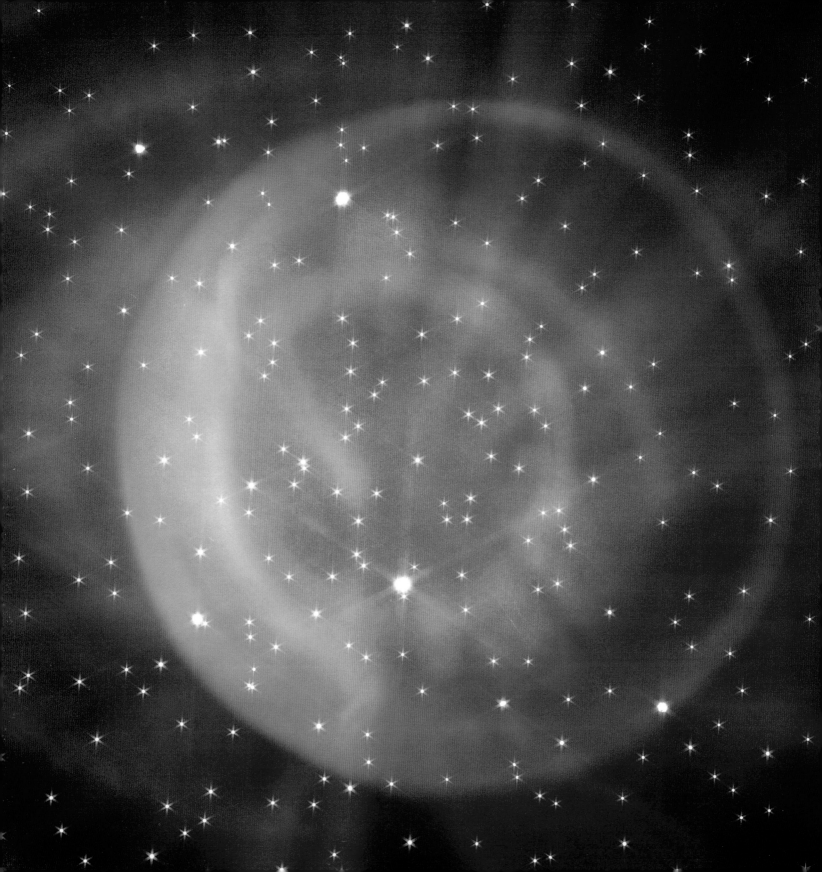

Part I
Your True Colors

Color Energy: The Bare Essentials

There is a Hopi creation myth that describes the rainbow—seven colored spears emerging out of black, stretching across and wrapping around our universe—as the first "thing" to ever exist. We now know the Hopis' vision of a universe made of color was not far off. The colors of a rainbow are composed of energy vibrating at seven different frequencies. These seven frequencies have been found to exist in particular energy centers of our bodies. So in a sense the Hopis were right—color is everything, color is what we're made of.

As the sun rises, its rays reveal a world resplendent with color. A single ray of sunshine contains all the colors of the spectrum. Yet the individual colors we see depend upon which of the sun's rays are absorbed by our surroundings and which are reflected. A red blanket, for instance, absorbs all the rays except for red, which are bounced back to our eyes, where the energy waves for red stimulate the light-sensitive cones in the retina; these in turn emit electrical impulses to the brain—and we see the red blanket. A blade of grass absorbs all the colors except green. The sky is blue or purple or gray depending on the absorption and reflection of particles in the air. Objects that appear white reflect all wave lengths, and black objects reflect none.

You Have an Aura About You

Scientists now accept that the energy of the sun is propelled through space in the form of electromagnetic waves, many of which are invisible to us. The waves that are visible are perceived as light, and when they bounce off everything around us, our earthly universe comes alive with color.

Human beings emit their own electromagnetic waves—as do all living (and even inanimate) things. Most of us already sense that we give off energy. When we say, "you have an aura about you," or that someone has bad vibes, sexy vibes, good vibes, we are referring to the energy field or "aura." Mystics and intuitives have frequently reported that they perceive the auras that surround us as fields of color. In fact, ever since antiquity, people have documented auras, whether they describe them as rays of light emanating from the body or as haloes or wings.

But most of us need more tangible evidence before we can accept the idea of auras, and in this day and age we have it. Scientists at UCLA and the University of Minnesota have confirmed that our aura consists of electromagnetic emanations that can actually be measured with the appropriate instruments. We saw the first graphic evidence in Kirilian, or high-voltage, photography. And several years ago a German researcher developed an Aura Video Station that allows you not only to see your aura but to watch its flow and vibrations on a monitor.

The most extensive work in this area has been done at UCLA by Dr. Valerie Hunt. In 1977, she published what is known as the Rolf energy study, prepared for the Rolf Institute of Structural Integration in Boulder, Colorado. Using a device known as an oscillator, Dr. Hunt successfully documented the existence of the human energy field, (also called the auric or bio field). Our aura usually extends about six to twelve inches out from our bodies, though the distance can be as great as four feet. (Yogis have been known to have auras that extend as far as a hundred feet.) Though few of us are able to see auras, it is important to understand that our bodies do extend beyond our skin.

Like fingerprints, auras are unique to each individual, and they interact with

For thousands of years, philosophers have debated the origin of color. Aristotle believed all colors were a blend of "darkness and lightness . . . Black mixed with sunlight and firelight turns crimson," he wrote. It was Sir Isaac Newton, in the seventeenth century, who discovered that color is a function of light.

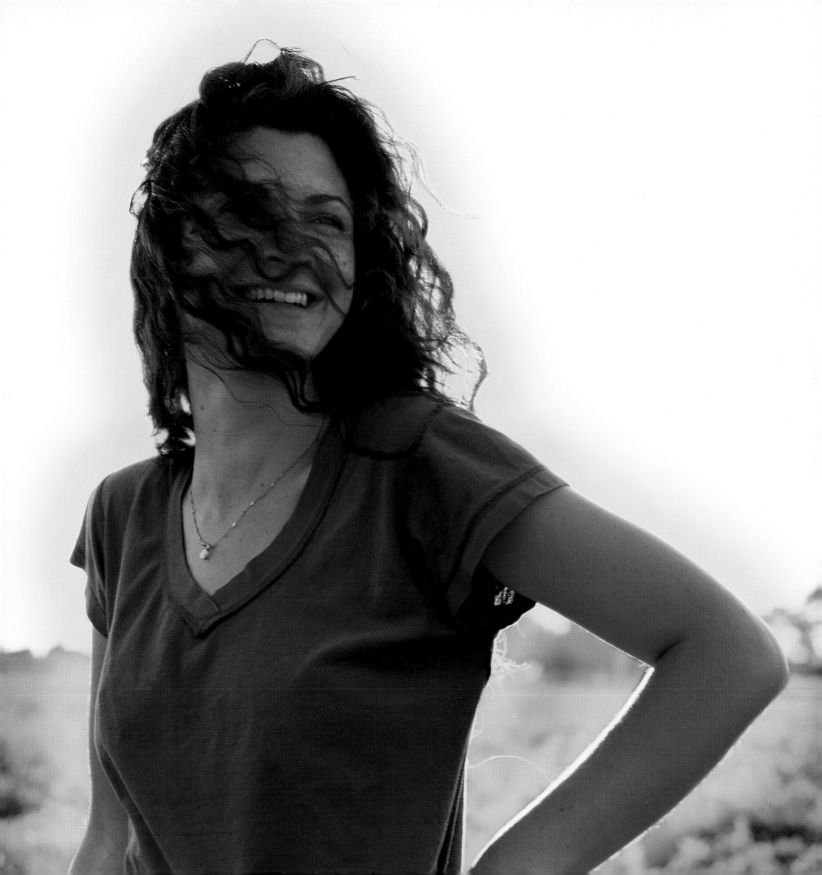

**HOW TO MEASURE YOUR
AURIC FIELD**

**Rub your hands together to
warm them. This helps you
sense the subtle energies of
your aura. Extend your arms
fully, hands facing each other,
as though you are holding a big
present for yourself. Slowly
move your hands toward each
other until you feel a slight
resistance between them. From
your hand to the center point is
how far your aura extends from
your body.**

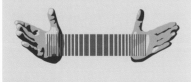

the auric fields of others. The longer and more intimate our contact with some-one, the greater the auric energy exchange will be. Contemporary healers tell us that the size and brightness of the aura reveals our mental, physical, emotional, and spiritual health at any given moment. The bigger and brighter, the better.

How do you know if your aura is strong? Your auric field is reflected in your overall health and ability to lead a happy, successful, and positive life. When your aura is weak, you literally become more porous, and outside forces more easily affect you. You may have trouble setting boundaries with others and may become tired easily.

What weakens the auric field?
- Drugs and alcohol
- Negative thought patterns such as anger and depression
- Poor diet
- Stress

What strengthens the auric field?
- Being in nature
- Sunshine
- Mind/body exercise
- Meditation
- Positive visualization
- Vibrational remedies

When we are aware of our personal aura, we can begin to understand why we're susceptible to the subtle energies both within and around us and why we are affected by them. And we can begin to understand the metaphysical ideas of the Egyptians and other early peoples, who believed that human health and behavior are influenced by the energy of color and by the planets, the rays of light reflected from gems, and the scents from plants.

The Chakras

The aura originates in the body's seven energy centers. Ancient Vedic texts identify these seven internal vortexes of energy as chakras—meaning, literally, "spinning wheels of light"—each of which is represented by a different color of the spectrum. Other cultures have similar constructs to describe these energy centers. The Tibetans identified six, each with a corresponding color. Straw dolls dating to pre-Egyptian times have been discovered with seven circles drawn on their forms that correspond to the Hindu energy centers. In the Jewish mystical writing known as Cabala there are seven centers of cosmic energy running the length of the human spine and extending through the skull. The oral tradition of the Hopi Indians tells of seven energy centers, each assigned a color of the spectrum ranging from red to white.

And now Dr. Hunt's study confirms the existence of the seven energy centers that correspond to the chakra centers described in Vedic texts.

Each internal chakra is an active vortex of energy that extends to the surface of the body. (This is how each center is connected to the aura.) Dr. Hunt found that the electromagnetic waves emanating from these centers exactly matched the frequencies of the colors of the spectrum associated with them. In that magical moment, modern science was finally united with ancient theories of native American and Eastern cultures.

There are seven major chakras within the human body and three that exist outside the physical body (one above and two below). There are also numerous secondary chakras in the joint areas of the feet, ankles, knees, hips, shoulders, neck, and hands, but it's the seven main chakras that we will focus on here.

Each of the seven chakras plays a role in the physical aspects of our being. Each is connected to a nerve plexus and major endocrine gland center. As energy is distributed through the spinal fluid to the nervous system, it moves into the chakras and out into the aura. Our bodies and chakras are one, so any malfunction of the chakras affects the whole endocrine system.

Each chakra also has its own emotional or spiritual aspect as well. Be-

HOW TO MASSAGE THE AURA

Massaging the aura by spinning in circles is one of five Tibetan exercises in the yogic tradition used to energize life force.

1. Stand with your arms hanging loosely at your sides and focus on a fixed point in front of you. Begin spinning around as you did when you were a child, turning clockwise. Each time you make a complete turn, bring your focus back to a fixed point on the wall in front of you. Try to spin a minimum of eleven times but no more than twenty-one. If you become too dizzy, stop. With practice, you will be able to do this exercise for longer periods.

2. After spinning, lie down. You'll notice that you'll continue to feel spinning sensations. This is fine. Go deeper and you'll feel your life force surging with energy.

cause the body and mind are inextricably joined, each chakra is not only linked to a specific area of the body but also to specific life issues. It might be said that each chakra affects a particular part of the mind, or as Rosalyn Bruyere writes, "has a mind of its own." In this way our chakras are keyholes that allow us to look into ourselves and understand why we behave as we do. Once we understand the chakras, we can understand our lives with the clarity and insight of a sage.

As we develop, our outlook is "colored" by specific chakras at different times of our lives. In childhood we're most strongly affected by the first chakra, located at the base of the spine; in later life we're influenced more by the seventh chakra, at the crown of the head. One by one, each chakra affects our point of view, our attitudes, and our behavior. But no chakra acts alone; each one is influenced by the others.

In the literature on the chakras you will find universal agreement on the colors of the first five chakras and then divergence of opinion on the last two. Some associate the sixth chakra with indigo and the seventh chakra with violet. The Hopi Indians, among others, referred to the sixth chakra as violet and the seventh as white. Since the Hindu word for the seventh chakra, Sahasrara, means "one with everything" and a rejoining with the source, and white is made up of a combination of the wave lengths of all colors, this makes sense to us. It also makes scientific sense. Dr. Hunt found that the people in her study who had balanced chakras emitted violet and white electromagnetic waves from their sixth and seventh chakras.

When the amount of energy that is generated by our seven chakras is strong, we experience well-being and health. When it becomes weak or out of balance, we experience malaise or illness. But we can learn to realign the chakras by using vibrational remedies, and few affect our energy system as powerfully as color. It is of us. Color therapy can benefit the specific physical, emotional, mental, and metaphysical qualities of the chakras and have a lasting effect on our general welfare.

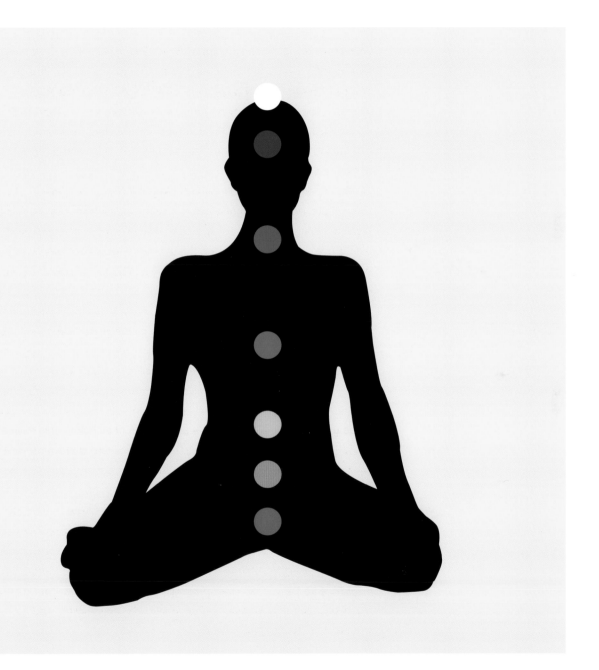

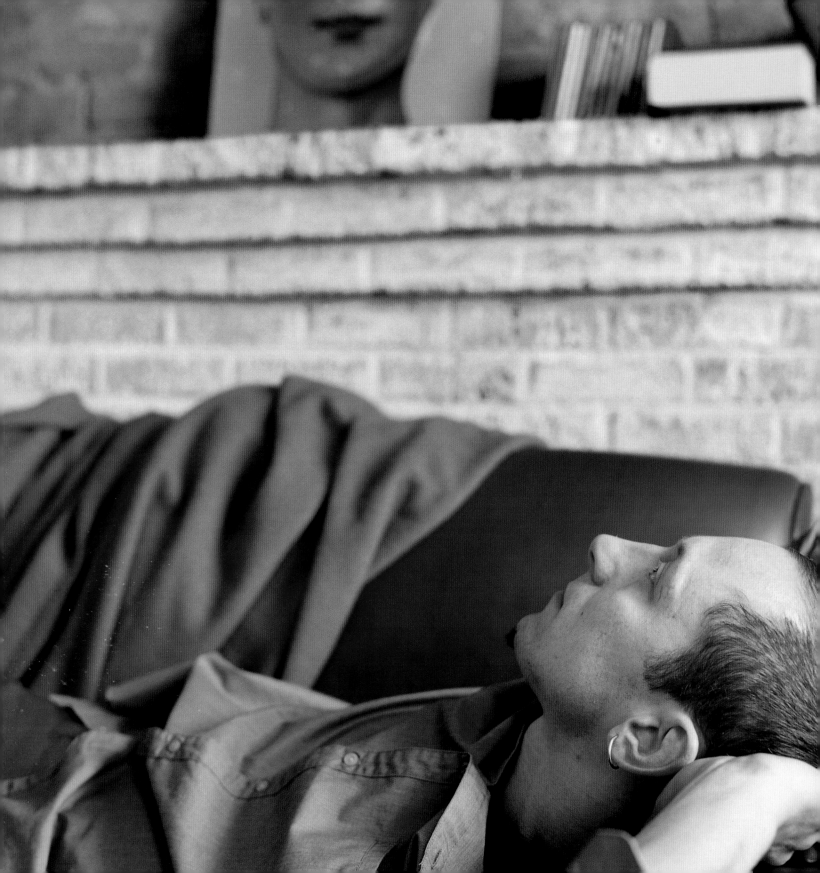

Finding Out What Colors You Need

How do you know which chakra is out of balance? How do you know which colors you lack and which you have too much of? Using color cards and/or the pendulum are simple ways to find out just which colors will help.

How We Began Our Color Card Readings

Personal appearances at cosmetic counters are a big part of our work, but early on we learned that spending our time painting nails while discussing the significance of the chakras didn't do much for our customers. Then we read about an exercise for healers in Ted Andrews's book *How to Heal with Color*, designed to teach healers to sense subtle energies and identify colors via flash cards. Necessity being the mother of invention, we adapted this technique for our customers, using color cards to identify weaknesses in chakra energy. We made color cards and printed the chakra associations on the back of each one. Then we asked our customers to close their eyes, move one hand over the cards, and note which cards produced the strongest sensation in their palms. This technique quickly indicated the colors they needed and, by extension, the chakras and corresponding life issues in need of attention.

People were fascinated with this process, and as we learned more, we began to give in-depth readings. The accuracy of our readings surprised no one more than us. It seemed that we were consistently identifying core issues, and often, when we did, powerful emotions instantly rose to the surface. Since most of us suppress the tough stuff, tears became a common sight in the cosmetics department.

Over the past five years we have done hundreds of these readings. We keep refining what Tina now calls our "home-grown diagnostic." Because of the cyclical nature of our store visits we occasionally see the same people six months to a year later, and they often tell us the color card reading was a catalyst to amazing transformations.

Doing Your Own Color Card Reading

You'll need seven cards that correspond to the seven chakras: red, orange, yellow, green, blue, purple, and white. Tony uses small cards, about the size of business cards; Cristina likes big ones the size of index cards, but any size will do. We painted our cards with acrylics because we had them around and they dry quickly. But if you don't have paints in the house or don't want to make your own cards, you can use the color cards printed in the back of this book, each with its chakra meaning on the back. Cut out the color cards and take them to a copy place to be laminated so they'll be durable and easy to use.

Once you have your cards, you're ready to begin. If you can, corral someone sympathetic to what you're doing to help. This can even be a child. But it's fine to do it alone. You can also do this process with friends and family.

1. Shuffle the cards and spread them out in front of you. They can be in one long row, slightly overlapping, or in two rows.

2. Close your eyes and rub your hands together for a few minutes until you feel a warmth between your palms.

3. Breathe deeply, then, using either your right or left hand, move your hand about two inches over the cards. If you have a helper, ask that person to see that your hand is over the cards and not hovering over something else. Take your time.

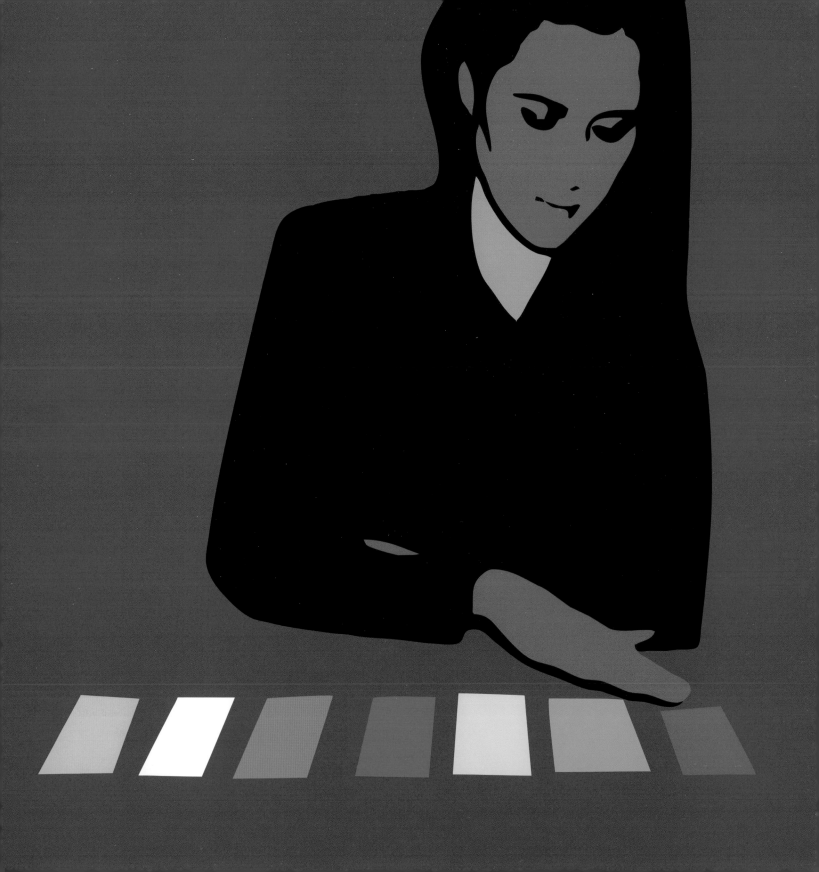

4. Concentrate as you move your hand over the cards; you will begin to feel a buzzlike sensation in your palm from one or two of the cards. Or you may sense a pull or a slightly heavy or hot feeling. People describe the sensation differently, so just listen to that gut feeling. You might even feel as though you're guessing. This is fine. Your unconscious is doing the work.

5. If you are drawn by two cards, note which has the stronger pull. Hold your hand over the cards you're responding to.

6. Open your eyes to see which cards you've chosen. Note which chakra the color card is related to. If you were drawn to two cards, the one from which you felt the strongest pull is your main life process right now; the other is secondary.

When you do a color reading for yourself, you will be amazed at the results. What could easily be considered a guessing game delivers uncanny feedback about your current state of mind. We've discovered that people with the same issues or concerns pick the same colors with remarkable consistency. Even if you feel as if you have made an arbitrary choice, trust that your internal wisdom has led you to the right card. Trust that your body knows what color it needs, just as it craves orange juice when you need vitamin C. Sometimes we're drawn to a color that relates to a difficult issue, but know that your consciousness wouldn't have led you there unless you were ready to deal with it.

As you think about the significance of your color card choices, consider both your deep-seated concerns as well as the more transitory issues. For instance, if I had a major unresolved problem such as the need to really forgive someone, I would be drawn to green. But if I just had a tense day and needed to relax I would also need green. Or perhaps I regretted the way I ignored a coworker all day; this would also prompt me to pick green. In assessing your color needs, play with your situation until you arrive at conclusions that feel right, just as you might with a dream about the day's events that also points to a deeper message from your psyche. If you're stumped by what the color cards might be telling you, check them for several days in a row to see if you are consistently drawn to one color. If that's the case, you are very likely ready to work on that area.

We discuss the meanings of the colors throughout the book, but for instant reference, see the meanings on the backs of the cards on page 159.

Using a Pendulum

You can also use a pendulum to help you determine which color energy you need. Pendulums have been used for centuries to ask the universe for answers to yes or no questions. To use a pendulum for color assessment, write the names of the seven colors of the spectrum an inch apart on a piece of paper, then hold the pendulum over each word or color.

A pendulum can be made from any object that dangles from a string, thread, or chain. You can buy a pendulum or make your own using almost anything— a fishing weight, a cork, a cross. We have found that quartz crystal pendulums work best because the quartz is a great transmitter of energy and can be programmed for specific tasks. It's smart energy. Besides asking your pendulum about your color needs, you can ask about illnesses, blockages, love or work problems, or even what to have for dinner. We consult the pendulum often.

The first step in using your pendulum is to assess which movement indicates a yes answer and which a no.

1. Spend a few minutes in deep breathing.

2. Gently but firmly hold the string of your pendulum so that the tip of the object is a few inches above a tabletop.

3. Holding the pendulum steady, ask it which direction will be yes. After a brief time, you will notice that although you are not moving the string, the pendulum has slowly begun to move. Despite your efforts to keep the pendulum still your unconscious is sending messages to your muscles and nerves causing the pendulum to move. The movement will be either clockwise, counterclockwise, back and forth in front of you, or side to side. When the pendulum has indicated which direction will be yes, ask it to indicate which direction will be no. The pendulum will answer with distinct movements for yes and no.

4. Now hold your pendulum over each color on your paper and find out what color you need.

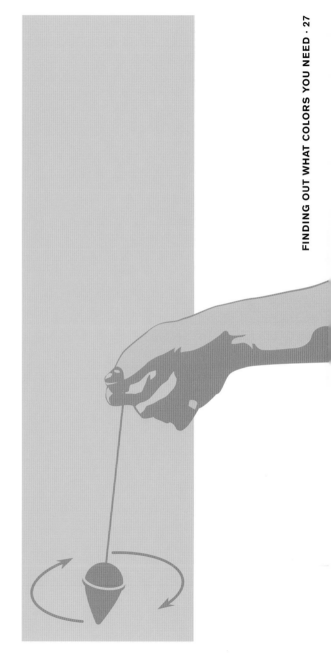

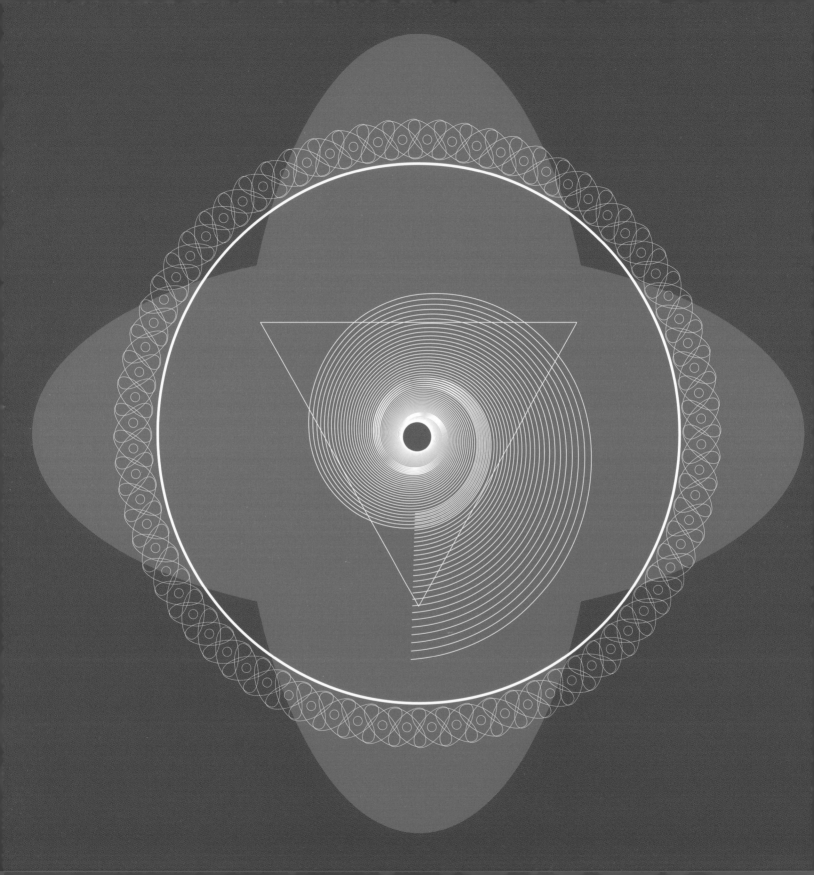

Red: The Body

element: fire / planet: mars / sign: scorpio / crystal: garnet / gemstone: ruby / essential oil: oakmoss / main life lessons: connect to parents, tribe; survive; procreate

Red is associated with the first chakra, also known as the root chakra, the energy center located at the base of the spinal column. Electromagnetic vibrations emitted by the color red exactly match the electromagnetic frequencies emitted from the root chakra. These frequencies are the lowest of all vibrations emitted from the seven chakras.

This energy center is associated with fire, the genitals, and our regenerative capacity; it literally gives us our fire power. The ancients understood it as the center of our primal life force, where our survival instincts are found. **It's the source of our vitality, leadership, strength, courage, and will.** It is related to the physical body and to male energy (some theorists relate it to female energy as well) and is associated with belonging to parents, grandparents, and to a people. This strong primal energy connects us all.

When your first chakra is balanced, you feel alive and at home in your own skin, in your family, in your community, and in the world. You feel a strong connection to your own body and to other people. You feel protected, are confident that your basic needs will be fulfilled and that things will somehow work out for you. When this center is blocked—when there is an interruption in

"Red. Red. Red. To ask a Latin girl for her favorite color is like asking Prince if he fancies purple. Red embodies guts. Red is the color of blood, of ripe tomatoes, of teasing (bullfighting), of danger signs, and of red-light districts. Pastels are a joke to us."

–*Jauretsi*

the natural flow of subtle energy through your system—you feel disconnected, alienated from others, and aggressive. You may have severe mood swings.

We all have base chakra issues to resolve about security, family, and belonging. Family ties are strong but so are family troubles. To experience the optimum power of the first chakra, we must resolve and heal family strife. In our work with the color cards we often find that people who select the red card complain of irrational fears. These fears come from feeling disconnected to the world, from feeling out on a limb.

We all need to examine the beliefs and behaviors that were passed on to us and then to consciously decide which we need to exorcize and which we want to keep. One friend who grew up in a home with overly critical parents has to learn to stop denigrating herself. She chose red during a color card reading because she needs to deal with red issues and learn to treat herself the way she always wanted to be treated. She needs to ask herself whether she wants to own the habit of self-criticism or trade it in for something else— something like self-love, which will lead to more inner peace. Using red will help her.

Our instincts are there to guide us. If there is something going on in your life that isn't making you feel good, then you need to summon up some red energy and do something about it. We have to stop blaming our adult failings on our childhood and take responsibility for who we are as adults. Working on base chakra issues can help everyone not only resolve family problems but help the other chakra centers function effectively.

Red chakra issues aren't just about the nuclear family; they include the family that forms within all kinds of groups, from sports teams to corporations. Breaking away from a corporation is often as difficult as leaving home.

A Red Color Card Reading with Tina

A woman marches up to my table with a serious expression on her face and sits down. As her hand scans the cards, it immediately hovers over red. Some people are drawn to two cards during a reading, but there was no questioning this woman's commitment to red. Her hand stops twice directly over the center of the card as if her eyes are open. I tell her that when you are drawn to this area you need to reevaluate the family traits you have retained as an adult. She smiles and nods. She tells me she's making big changes in her life but doesn't say what they are. I say I guess I should mention red energy also has to do with personal safety issues and standing up for yourself. Her eyes fill with tears and she tells me that her husband has abused her physically and emotionally for many years and that she has finally left him.

When this woman summoned up her courage and left her husband, she drew from her primal instinct for self-protection—red energy. She tells me that she had begun to be attracted to red around the time she finally realized she had had enough. She began to buy red things for the house, pillows, a new lipstick, and so forth. She instinctively knew she needed the red energy to take action and stick with her resolve. As an afterthought, she says she had a family history of abuse. Many women like her are taught in nonverbal ways that it's okay to be abused. I tell that with her action—her refusal to take it—she has stopped the cycle—that it is said that if you truly heal, you not only heal yourself but the seven generations to come.

If you find yourself drawn to red, one of two things is usually happening. First, there might be a family situation or inherited trait that's giving you trouble. Make sure no family beliefs are blocking your personal expression. Second, you need to explore your fears, especially the fear of the future and/or death or for your personal safety. Use the red energy to support you in working through these two processes. Face them without expectation but with faith for yourself, and you will always be on the right path.

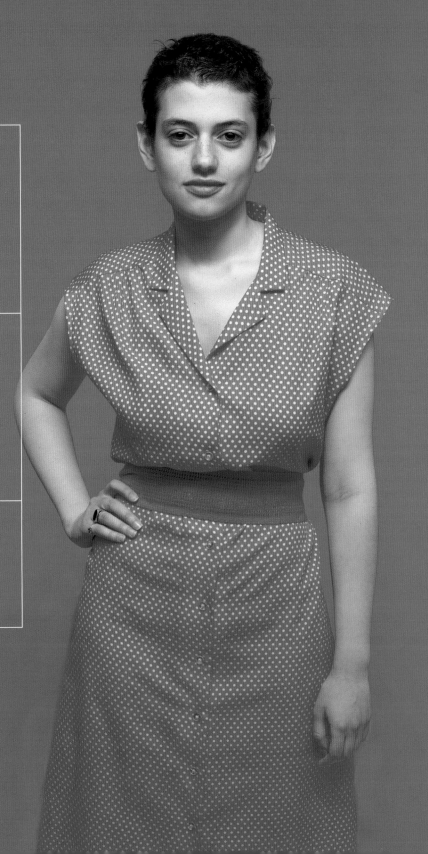

Red Issues

If you have too much red you:
- Aggressively act out
- Have trouble sleeping
- Are egotistic
- Are domineering
- Are greedy
- Use sexual energy indiscriminately

To balance, use green followed by
a small amount of red.

If you have too little red you:
- Depend on outside belief systems to
  justify your actions
- Lack confidence
- Feel weak
- Feel fearful
- Are self-destructive
- Have a fear of being abandoned

You need more red.

When you have just enough red you are:
- Centered
- Grounded
- Healthy
- Can manifest abundance
- Have unlimited physical energy

The Red Period of Our Relationship

 The first real risk I ever took was when I quit my corporate job. It was very much a first-chakra issue. I had done what most Gen-Xers do in their twenties. I had passively protested my family's and my corporation's way of doing things but I was still playing the game. I was losing my personal integrity, and I had to make a change. I had to form a family with myself, create a new set of beliefs based on my own experiences, decide how I wanted to live my life. Leaving a nice predictable paycheck and colleagues I liked was a bit like walking the plank. It was the red energy of the base chakra that gave me the drive to do it.

Once I made the decision to leave, the universe seemed ready to support me. I met Tony, and he showed me new possibilities about how I could be. He took my ideas and talents seriously and gave me courage and a sense of groundedness. I believe that you are instinctively drawn to people of your own soul group; when you meet them, your bond becomes strong quickly because you are already bonded on the spiritual level. Tony and I are family. I am very fortunate to have him. He continues to be a constant source of love and support in my life. My tribal ties to him are endless and beginningless.

I met Cristina at a party in 1995. I was this English guy at this New York party full of swanky, uptown American girls. It was my last weekend on the trip. I felt kind of fateful. And then at some point the doorbell rang and Cristina walked in looking, in her words, very shleppy. She had this huge sweater on and hair like she'd been in bed for a week. She had a black eye and she looked slightly jaundiced. The juxtaposition of these uptown girls all dressed in Donna Karan and Cristina looking like Our Gang . . . We started talking and she had an incredible attitude about her. She'd just recovered from mono and she'd gotten her black eye from being elbowed in the pit of a Hole gig. She had no intention of coming to the party, but something drove her to get out of her sick bed and come.

We really did fall in love that night. The beginning of our relationship was

RED FACTOIDS

Red has carried powerful meanings and symbolism for peoples and cultures throughout history. The associations are often contradictory–red usually carries the connotations of love and procreation, but it is also associated with violence and death. Although meanings can vary between and within cultures, in general it can be said that red is most often connected with our most primal instincts, procreation and aggression.

In ancient Egypt, the color red was the color of the hostile god Sutech and was associated with violence.

By contrast, in China, during the Chou dynasty, red was considered a sacred and vitalizing color. Brides still traditionally wear red in the Chinese marriage ceremony to bring good luck.

In the Christian tradition, red is the color of the sacrificial blood of Christ, and the color of vestments worn by cardinals. But it also became known as the color of Hell and the Devil.

PINK

A mixture of white and red, pink is the color that represents love on the spiritual plane. It helps in attracting love and affection and can provoke the giddy feeling that often accompanies joy and laughter.

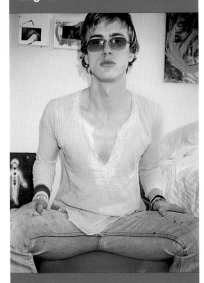

"My three favorite colors? Pink, pink, and *pink*! Several years ago I painted my New York apartment a bold pink—halfway between L.A. Barbie bubble-gum pink and Florida flea market coral. I've been totally tickled ever since!"
—*Audrey*

very much about the red chakra that gives you the power to manifest desires in the physical world. Meeting Cristina was like crossing a bridge. Like a big exhale.

Cristina's understanding of the spiritual realm excited and inspired me. We had both decided we were meant for great things and committed to help each other overcome our personal obstacles. About that time, I left London for good. I felt that I had to cut ties with my original tribe and leave a situation that couldn't take me any further. I wanted to find out just what I was capable of. Cristina became my new tribal family. Our union was very powerful. We felt unstoppable.

The exercise on the opposite page and the visualization below can be used to enhance the red energy in your body. In the following chapters, you'll find exercises designed for specific colors as well as general color exercises in Part 2, Feeding Yourself Color Energy (page 77).

Visualization

Take the shade off a table lamp and put in a red lightbulb. Sit for a few minutes in silence and breathe deeply. See yourself surrounded in red. Within this light you are strong, balanced, courageous, and safe in your own hands. Imagine standing up for yourself, strong, filled with energy and happiness. You are safe and comfortable in your own body. Breathe that image in.

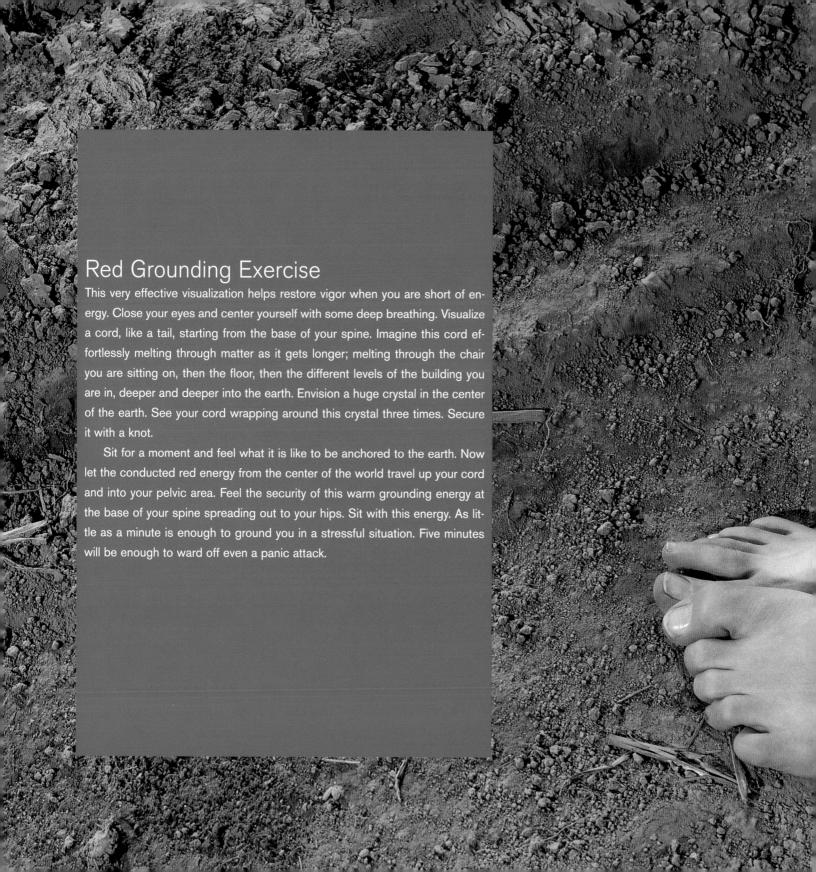

Red Grounding Exercise

This very effective visualization helps restore vigor when you are short of energy. Close your eyes and center yourself with some deep breathing. Visualize a cord, like a tail, starting from the base of your spine. Imagine this cord effortlessly melting through matter as it gets longer; melting through the chair you are sitting on, then the floor, then the different levels of the building you are in, deeper and deeper into the earth. Envision a huge crystal in the center of the earth. See your cord wrapping around this crystal three times. Secure it with a knot.

Sit for a moment and feel what it is like to be anchored to the earth. Now let the conducted red energy from the center of the world travel up your cord and into your pelvic area. Feel the security of this warm grounding energy at the base of your spine spreading out to your hips. Sit with this energy. As little as a minute is enough to ground you in a stressful situation. Five minutes will be enough to ward off even a panic attack.

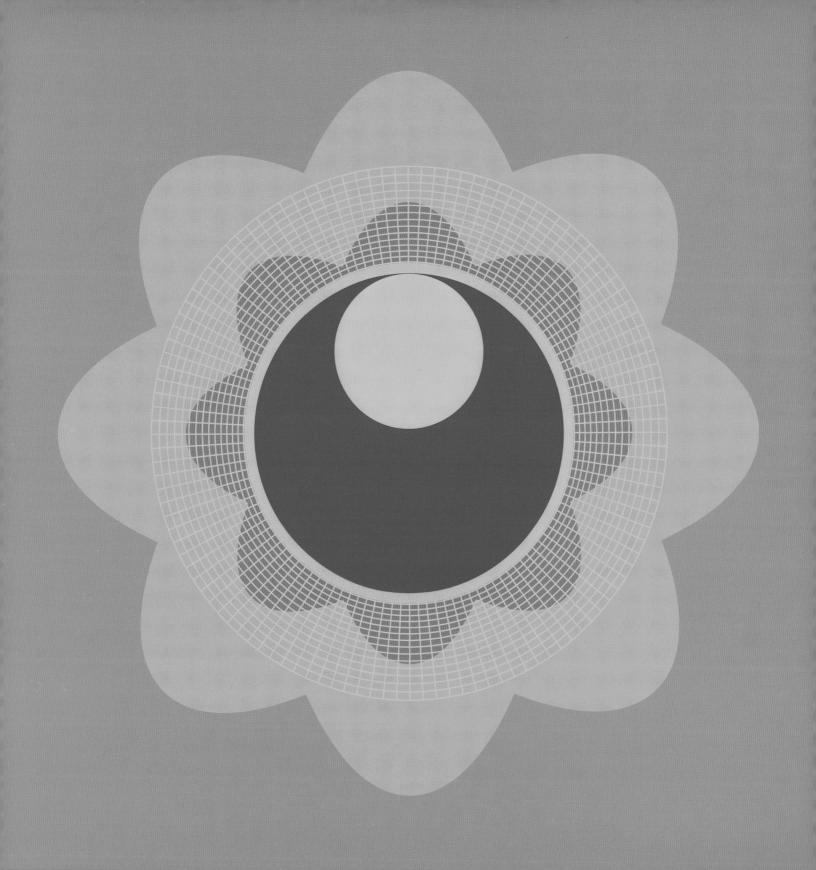

Orange: The Emotions

element: water / planet: moon / crystal: carnelian /
gemstone: pearl / essential oil: neroli / main life lessons:
connect to others; boundaries; sensuality; power

The electromagnetic vibrations emitted by orange exactly match the frequencies emitted from the second, or spleen, chakra. This chakra is located in the center of the abdomen between the red and yellow chakras. Just as orange is a mixture of red and yellow, so the orange chakra shares some of the traits of its neighbors. It governs instincts, desires, sexuality, feeling, and creative expression. **It is our power center, the seat of our emotions and intuition.** While the energy of the base red chakra allows us to feel secure and grounded in our community, the orange chakra energy allows us to move beyond the protection and constraints of the tribe and form partnerships outside our families.

It is in the orange center that we receive emotional guidance from our higher selves in the form of gut feelings. Because our families, community, society, and the media train us not to trust our gut, exploring this energy center can be tricky. Most of us aren't comfortable standing by our intuition and going against the tide, which is perhaps why so many people avoid this color. But our feelings and perceptions are our only true reality, so we must listen to our instincts. When we don't like what we hear, we can be sure it is an area we need to work on.

"I've really been into orange. . . . I have this orange lipstick and even though it's not the best color for me, I sometimes wear it or just take it out of my cosmetic bag to look at. It makes me feel better."

–Rebecca

Rebecca's in a new job and a new marriage, dealing with all the orange issues–sex, money, and power. She is instinctively feeding herself this specific orange energy during a time when she is negotiating her new role both at home and at work.

It's from this chakra that we register our appetites and the sensations of sound, touch, smell, sight, and taste. The orange chakra is our pleasure center, and when it is in balance we feel an excitement and exuberance about life. We are open to the myriad sensory stimuli surrounding us. We savor and enjoy. We can express our sexuality. We are in touch with our spontaneity, our intuition, our joy, and our creativity. Because this chakra is the source of our sensuality and self-expression, it attracts others to us. It is socially stimulating and we feel an easy connection and flow with those around us. When it is misaligned, we have problems with sexuality and boundaries, ethics, honor, and money. This chakra is the center of our desire to be what we were born to be.

The orange chakra is also our humor center, where laughter originates. When this center is balanced we are at ease, we are fluid, we are vital people. We exude a passion for life and effortlessly establish positive relations not only with our mates and lovers but with friends, relatives, colleagues. Our second chakra gives us the power to manifest all that we desire.

As children, our chakra centers are particularly sensitive. We are like sponges picking up the subtlest of energies, especially those related to our creativity and our sexuality. When our families value inventiveness and intuition, we develop with our sense of innovation and spontaneity intact. When our parents accept and celebrate sensuality, we feel free with our naked bodies. Negative parental attitudes can result in a legacy of sexual blockage that may be passed from generation to generation. In these cases, orange chakra issues need to be revisited and recharged.

An underactive orange chakra can cause sexual insecurity and repression. People with this problem may find themselves needy in their relationships, as well as guilt-ridden about sexual desire. They might also find themselves on the wrong side of power struggles at work.

An overactive orange chakra can cause an individual to be sexually indiscriminate and use sexual energy to manipulate others. Such a person may be quick to anger if rebuffed. Too much orange can also motivate people to manipulate others in more general ways.

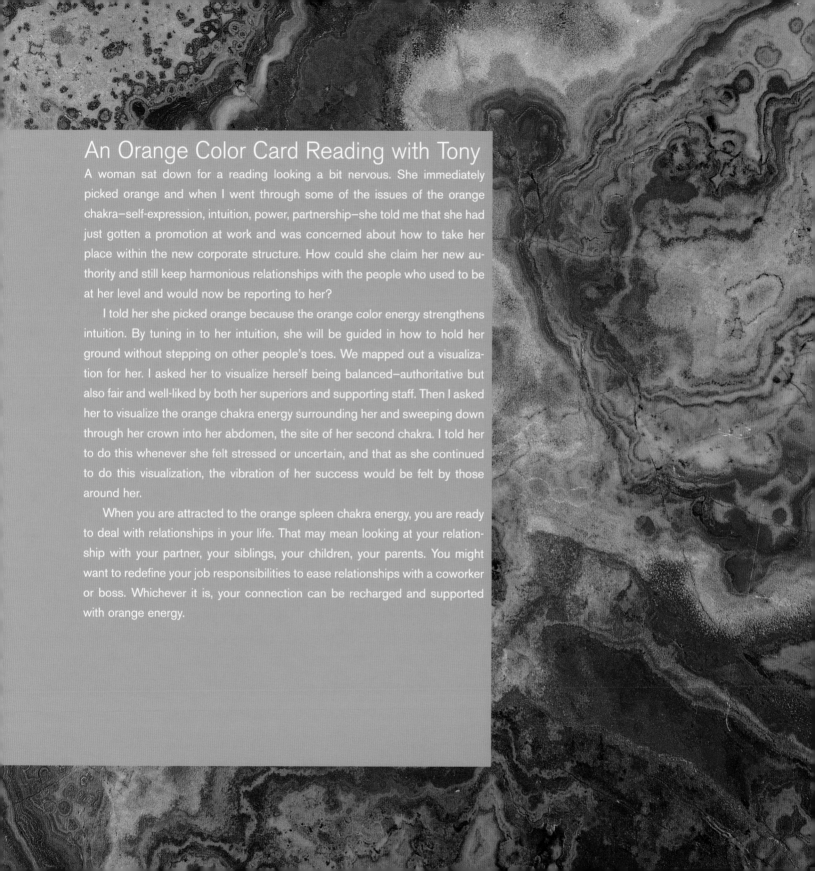

An Orange Color Card Reading with Tony

A woman sat down for a reading looking a bit nervous. She immediately picked orange and when I went through some of the issues of the orange chakra—self-expression, intuition, power, partnership—she told me that she had just gotten a promotion at work and was concerned about how to take her place within the new corporate structure. How could she claim her new authority and still keep harmonious relationships with the people who used to be at her level and would now be reporting to her?

I told her she picked orange because the orange color energy strengthens intuition. By tuning in to her intuition, she will be guided in how to hold her ground without stepping on other people's toes. We mapped out a visualization for her. I asked her to visualize herself being balanced—authoritative but also fair and well-liked by both her superiors and supporting staff. Then I asked her to visualize the orange chakra energy surrounding her and sweeping down through her crown into her abdomen, the site of her second chakra. I told her to do this whenever she felt stressed or uncertain, and that as she continued to do this visualization, the vibration of her success would be felt by those around her.

When you are attracted to the orange spleen chakra energy, you are ready to deal with relationships in your life. That may mean looking at your relationship with your partner, your siblings, your children, your parents. You might want to redefine your job responsibilities to ease relationships with a coworker or boss. Whichever it is, your connection can be recharged and supported with orange energy.

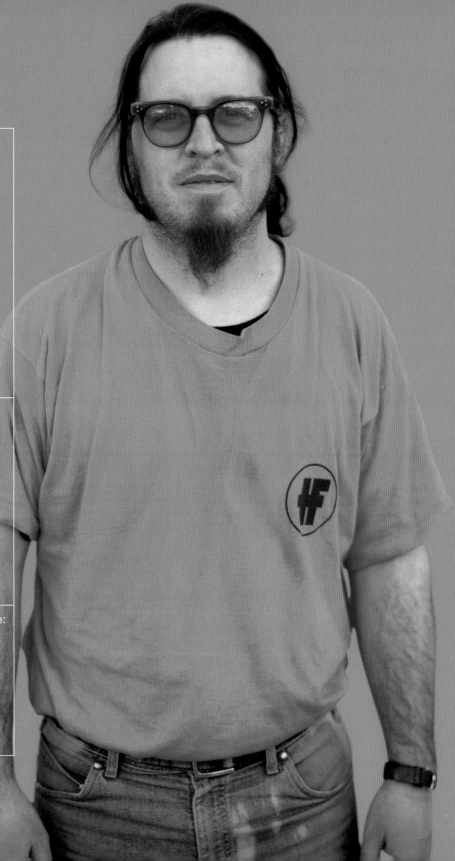

Orange Issues

Orange Issues

If you have too much orange you are:
- Emotionally explosive
- Aggressive
- Dominant in a relationship
- Prone to hyperactivity
- Manipulative
- Overindulgent
- Obsessed with sex
- Overambitious
- Likely to see people as sex objects

If you have too much orange you need blue followed by a small amount of orange.

If you have too little orange you are:
- Likely to have an imbalance of power within a relationship regarding sex, money, or power
- Resentful
- Sensitive
- Prone to feelings of guilt
- Prone to sexual blocks
- Distrustful
- Not open with your feelings

When you have just enough orange you are:
- Friendly
- Optimistic
- Creative
- Caring
- Intuitive
- Connected to your feelings

Our Orange Period: We're in Love

Once Tony and I had bonded on a tribal level we settled into our true partnering. I believe this can happen only when the sexual panic ends. In the beginning of a relationship you want to get as close to the other person as fast as possible, and our physical instincts drive us to engage in high levels of sexuality. It's a very exciting and overwhelming time for two people in love, consumed by the fire of red chakra energy. But as the relationship progresses, the desperation subsides and you get on with the business of becoming an "us" and a "we." This is where you develop roles as a couple. But no matter what stage your relationship is in, your role will always shift again, so you'll want to revisit this chakra. Change is unbelievably beautiful once you accept that it is a constant. With every breath we have the ability to be reborn.

At this point Tony and I decided to become each other's fuel for life. We spent days and nights on end playing with ideas of who we were and what we could do.

In the orange period of our relationship, our encouragement of each other really turned on the taps of creativity. We made a lot of paintings and a lot of plans. In many ways, our exploration of each other led us to know ourselves on a deeper level. Our union was very powerful. Actually, we spent more time laughing than anything else.

Cristina opened me to a new level of honesty different from any other relationship I had known. She made me feel safe enough to realize that I was so preoccupied with the idea of what sex should be that I spent the whole time in the third person, as it were, observing and nearly missing out on the whole experience. Cristina was the only person I had met who was self-aware enough to teach me that there was more to sex than my preconceived macho model. The implications of this discovery moved far beyond sex. I was beginning my quest to become present at all times.

ORANGE FACTOIDS

Tibetan Buddhist monks have long worn orange as a sign of wisdom. Spontaneity, intuition, living in the present moment—all orange chakra characteristics—are also fundamental Buddhist precepts. The Hari Krishna Hindu sect wears orange robes for similar reasons.

In China and Japan, orange is thought to symbolize joy and happiness.

An ex–football star told us that some sports managers are well aware of the power of color and use it to manipulate energy. When he visited Atlanta on the guest team, the players were given locker rooms painted black, gray, and dull shades of purple—colors specifically intended to deflate morale. Years later, returning to Atlanta as a new member of the home team, he found orange and yellow locker rooms with red neon lights and loud, upbeat music. The home team instantly pumped up and began the battle before they even got on the field!

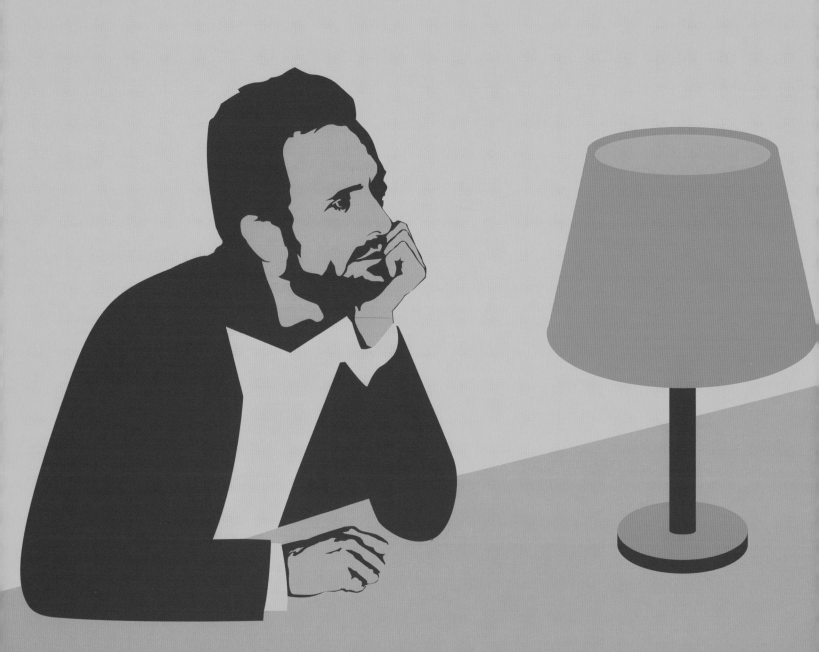

ORANGE: THE EMOTIONS · 43

Visualization

Sit for a few minutes in a quiet room (or wherever you happen to be) and breathe deeply. See yourself submerged in a beautiful orange light. You are connected to your inner wisdom and it guides all of your emotion and actions. You are capable of resolving any and all situations effectively. You are comfortable with power and sexuality. Breathe that in.

Meditation with an Orange Lightbulb

Put an orange lightbulb in a table lamp and leave the shade on. Sit quietly and absorb the orange energy for eight minutes. The orange energy will either relax or stimulate you, depending on your color needs. If you wish, you can also use an orange cloth draped over the lampshade instead of the lightbulb.

What to think about under orange light: It is the nature of the orange center to flow with creativity. Allow this to happen. Affirm to yourself that you have an open channel to a deep inner wisdom. Think about how you treat the people closest to you. Affirm your wish to be good to others and that your relationships bring joy. Allow this orange energy to alleviate your need to control situations. Trust that your inner wisdom will always be there to guide you.

INTUITION

As enlightened beings, our intuition will always guide us the right choices. But since most of us are just beginning to connect with, and trust, our intuition, we may still need some practice. By continually testing what feels right, you will gradually learn to interpret your inner signals. Your instincts never steer you wrong.

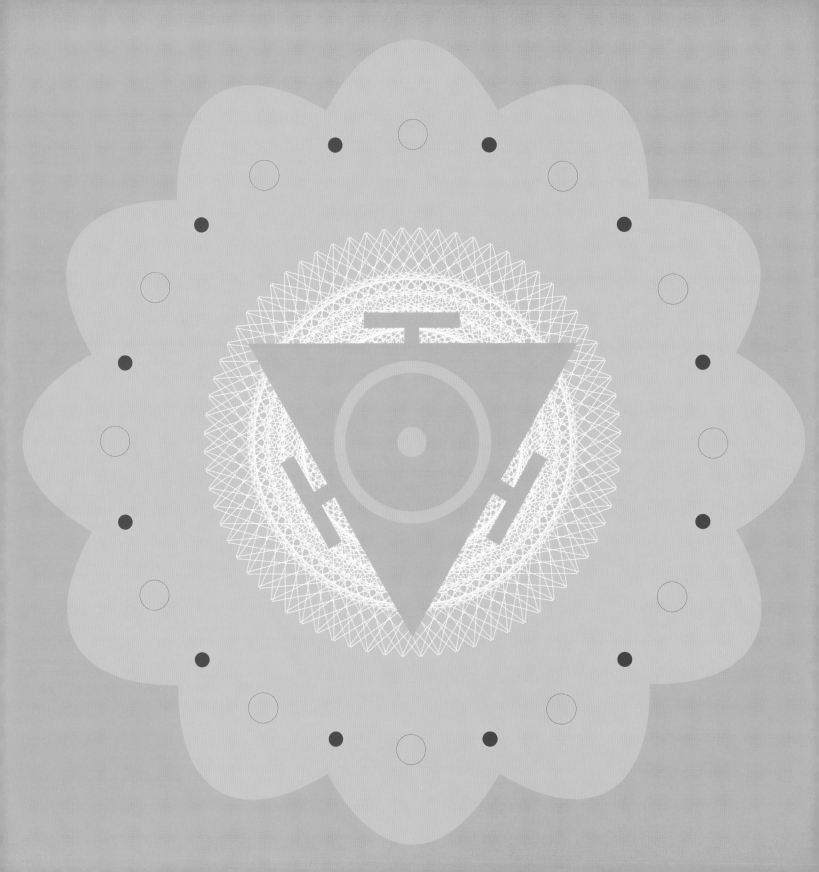

Yellow: The Intellect

element: air / planet: sun / sign: leo / crystal: heliodor /
gemstone: topaz / essential oil: bergamot / main life lessons:
inner power; self-esteem; self-acceptance

The electromagnetic frequency of the color yellow exactly matches the frequency of the third chakra, located in the solar plexus between the navel and the rib cage. This chakra is related to the adrenal glands and is the site of our intellectual and personal power as well as our sense of self. It is our command center, the place where our intention and will take shape, where our thoughts and opinions are formed. This center enables us to move forward toward the fulfillment of our desires and our goals.

The color yellow stimulates thought and allows us to exercise the intellectual and emotional force we need in order to make decisions and find our way. It also enables us to take the personal risks necessary so as to form attachments and develop close relationships with others. It is our second intuitive center (after orange); when fully developed, it reinforces our intellectual decisions and serves as a rudder as we chart our course in life.

The yellow energy of the solar plexus chakra supports our inner power and allows us to develop self-esteem. Although we project this self-esteem out to the world around us, it also plays a crucial role in our relationship with ourselves. The journey to inner power, with its constant peaks and valleys, is a

A Yellow and Violet Color Card Reading with Tina

A young girl of about fifteen or sixteen sat down for a color card reading and chose yellow and purple. When I heard her story, it wasn't hard to see why. She was recovering from anorexia, her self-esteem was on the mend, and she needed to view things objectively. Her therapist was unable to identify the underlying problem that drove her to starve herself. Had she been neglected? Abandoned? Abused? No, no, and no. In fact, there was no tangible problem and the girl sometimes wondered if she had the right to be sick.

In fact, the culprit here was society itself. When this young girl started dating, she developed this idea about what she should look like and how she should be. Thin was at the top of the list. Since her recovery, she has watched three of her friends follow the same pattern. The culprit wasn't their boyfriends or their peer group. It was society, which makes young girls and women feel they can never measure up to a physical ideal.

Our solar plexus chakra is especially vulnerable because it's the chakra that is most easily drained by other people. We are all so sensitive. Realizing that negativity from other people has a direct affect on us is the first step to protecting ourselves from energy downers. We need to nurture ourselves into a place where we see how wonderful we really are.

Violet energy of the third-eye chakra can be very helpful when used in conjunction with yellow energy. As you'll learn in later chapters, violet, or purple energy connects us with our extrasensory perception and helps us to see ourselves symbolically. It allows us to see our path clearly, deflect the negative messages, and recognize our true beauty. It is only our misperception of ourselves that stops us.

never-ending one. When the third chakra is aligned, it gives us the firm support we need for our self-esteem to grow and flourish.

You are attracted to yellow energy, just as with orange, when you need to have more trust in yourself. Trusting your instincts gives you an amazing sense of power and confidence. When you are dealing with self-esteem issues, it is important to consciously do things that will better your opinion of yourself. You will also need to evaluate the people and situations in your life that are draining you of positive energy and take action accordingly.

A Yellow Color Card Reading with Tony

A young woman sits down and I notice that she is unable to look me in the eye. Her hair falls over her cheek and hides half her face. Her shoulders are hunched and she nods tentatively when I explain what to do. With her eyes shut tight, she hovers over the cards. In a voice I can barely hear, she says "This one," and stops at the yellow card. We talk about self-esteem and she tells me she is the plain sister, that she has always been unpopular and lonely. I explain to her that the solar plexus chakra, where we hold our ideas about self, is often programmed by the negative messages we received as children that we play back to ourselves over and over. I tell her that we can reprogram this chakra by using a seven-night visualization (page 51). She writes down all the steps, brushes the hair out of her eyes, and gives me a big smile.

The Yellow Period of Our Relationship

 At this point we had begun to drain each other of yellow energy, something a lot of couples do. What happens is that your mental processes are stimulated in the third chakra, and you begin to challenge each other. Your intention is always good; you want to strengthen the relationship and you are trying to support your partner's goals by pushing. But the problem is that we all don't get to the other side of the road the same way. Being critical and pushy usually breeds resentment.

You are attracted to the yellow color energy when you need to have more trust in both yourself and in others close to you. Trusting your instincts gives you an amazing sense of power and confidence in yourself. (Your gut instinct, which originates in the orange chakra as an emotion, appears here in a more cerebral form.) This is a time to consciously do things that will better your opinion of yourself, and to be sensitive to how your words and actions are making others feel, particularly those very close to you. This is also the time to evaluate the people and situations in your life that might be draining you of this energy and make changes accordingly.

Unfortunately, this is what happened to Tony and me. At first we boosted each other's self-esteem sky high. Later, we became judgmental. We became disablers, and drained each other of inner power. Judgments are a destroyer of relationships. We were so depleted we didn't have the motivation to make all the positive changes we were so busily pointing out to each other, which left us to wallow and fight.

We really don't need to have so many opinions about each other. If our partner is doing something we don't like, we don't need to waste energy judging or being angry. As my dad always said, "It's easier to just say to yourself 'that's an interesting way to do things' and leave it."

Tony and I were not so good at leaving it. Neither of us let the other get away with a thing, and this struggle blocked our love. Finally, we broke up.

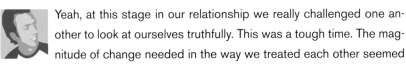 Yeah, at this stage in our relationship we really challenged one another to look at ourselves truthfully. This was a tough time. The magnitude of change needed in the way we treated each other seemed overwhelming. Although by this time the company was rolling along at a great pace, our self-esteem quotients were at all-time lows. We had both just turned thirty and we had a lot of stock-taking to do. We were constantly holding up a mirror to each other and we both made sure it only reflected the worst. Not a great time for us, but nothing happens without a reason.

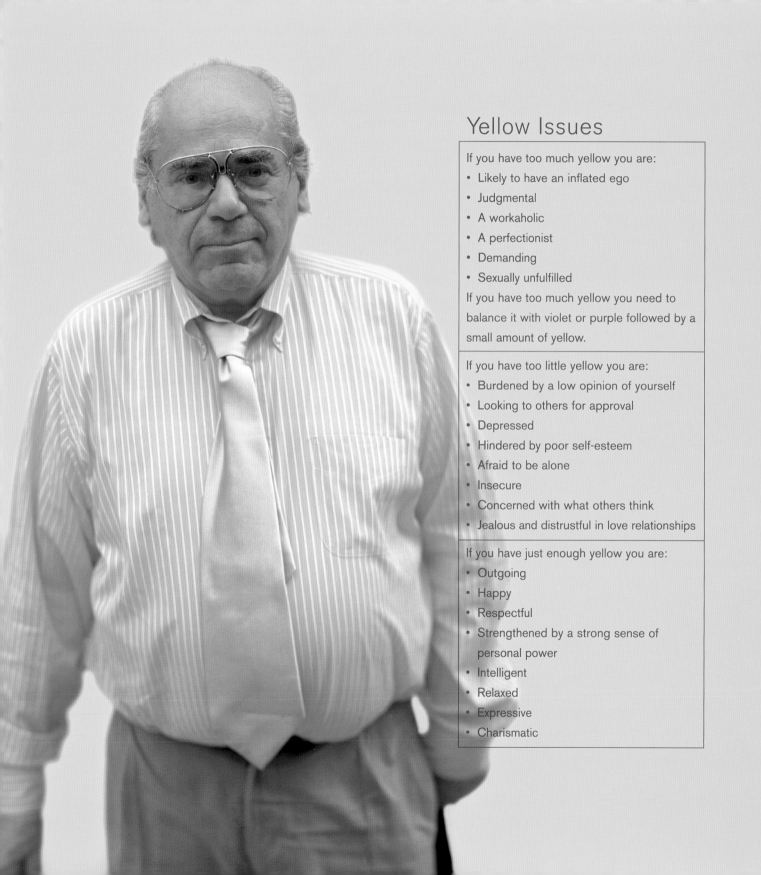

Yellow Issues

If you have too much yellow you are:
- Likely to have an inflated ego
- Judgmental
- A workaholic
- A perfectionist
- Demanding
- Sexually unfulfilled

If you have too much yellow you need to balance it with violet or purple followed by a small amount of yellow.

If you have too little yellow you are:
- Burdened by a low opinion of yourself
- Looking to others for approval
- Depressed
- Hindered by poor self-esteem
- Afraid to be alone
- Insecure
- Concerned with what others think
- Jealous and distrustful in love relationships

If you have just enough yellow you are:
- Outgoing
- Happy
- Respectful
- Strengthened by a strong sense of personal power
- Intelligent
- Relaxed
- Expressive
- Charismatic

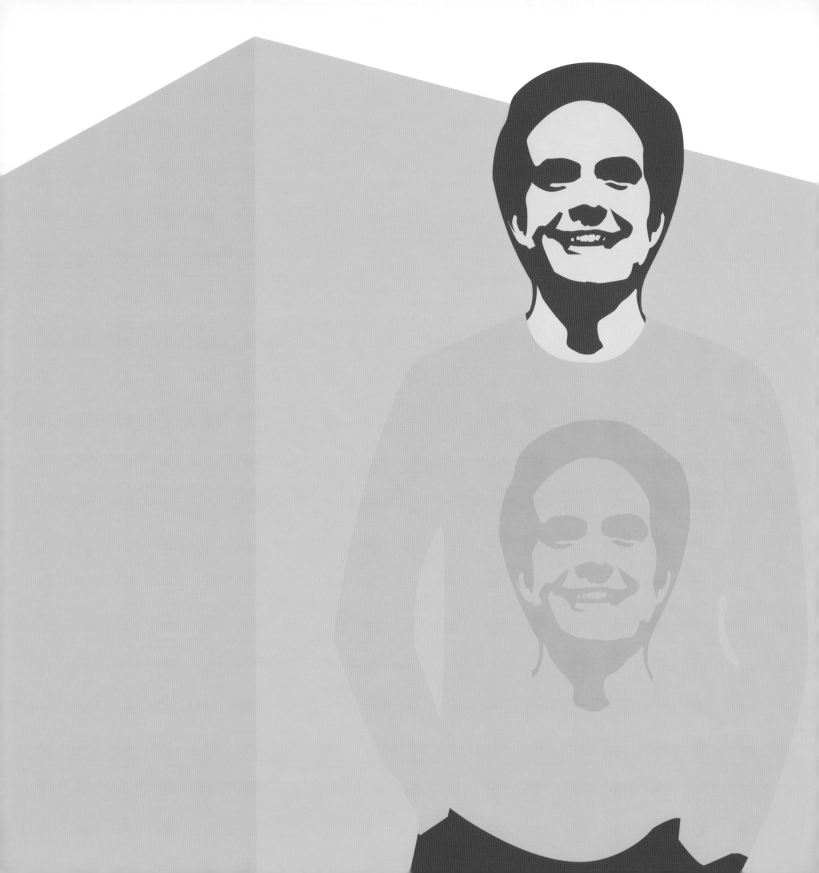

Yellow Chakra Reprogramming
(Seven-Night Visualization)

1. For one week, go to bed a little earlier than usual. Breathe deeply and concentrate on the yellow solar plexus chakra just above your navel, right below the rib cage. When you can see it in your mind's eye, imagine that you are traveling into this yellow light until you are in a sunshine-filled space deep within you.

2. In this space, see an image of yourself as a child playing. Introduce yourself and nurture this child as though it were your own. Ask him what he wants to be when he grows up. Tell her how beautiful she is, how clever, how compassionate, and so on.

3. Allow this visualization to continue as you drop off to sleep. This will open the realms of your subconscious to healing energy. As one of our teachers explained to us: Whatever we go to sleep thinking about is what our subconscious meditates on while we sleep. Falling asleep with negative thoughts just makes you wake up tired and grumpy. Going to sleep with positive images can aid your transformation to your ideal self.

4. Continue nurturing your child for the rest of the week. (The number seven has magical qualities.) This process will leave your yellow chakra positively reprogrammed and you will feel the change in your self-esteem immediately. Believe in it and allow it to be true.

Note: For an immediate confidence boost, you can also picture this chakra glowing with yellow light.

In early Greece and Rome, yellow (and red) were associated with love. But later, courtesans adopted yellow and it became the color associated with sensuality and promiscuity. Thus the early Christians viewed the color yellow with suspicion and it became associated with treachery. This continued up to sixteenth-century France, where the doors of traitors and criminals were smeared with yellow, and into the last century, when the yellow star, stitched to a coat, became a sign of damnation.

For the Moors, golden yellow signified wise and good counsel whereas pale yellow signified treachery and deceit. In heraldry, too, gold is an emblem of love, constancy, and wisdom. In our day, the bored lover signals the end of the affair by sending yellow roses. Yellow also carries the connotation of cowardly (The Cowardly Lion) or irresponsible behavior—as when a tabloid is accused of "yellow journalism." Gold, a symbol of money in our time, is also referred to as filth, as in "filthy lucre."

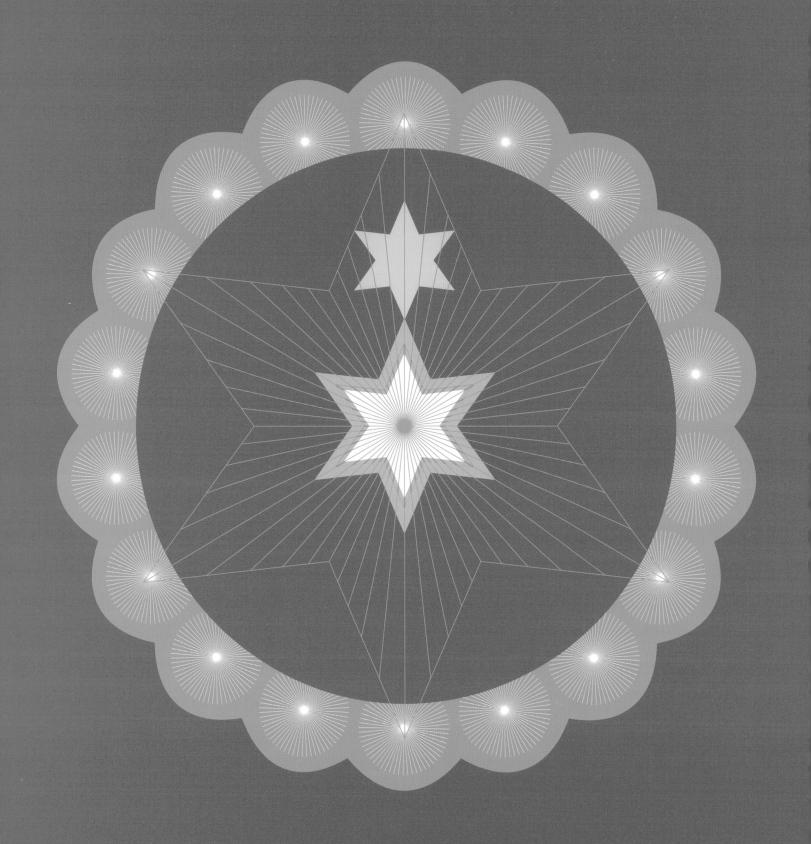

Green: The Heart

element: air / planet: venus / signs: taurus and libra /
crystal: green tourmaline / gemstone: emerald / essential oil: rose /
main life lessons: compassion and forgiveness

The frequency of green exactly matches the frequency of the fourth or heart chakra, located in the center of the chest near the heart and related to the thymus, a part of the lymph system. The heart chakra links the three physical chakras of the lower body to the three spiritual chakras in the upper body, merging matter and spirit. It is also where our male and female energies meet (see page 75 for male/female balancing exercise). When this center is balanced, we feel safe, able to trust, to love, to feel loved, to receive love, and to take risks. **When our heart chakra is balanced and open we are loving, kind, tolerant, and compassionate toward those around us.** Our tendency to be judgmental, to look for blame, and to be suspicious recedes as does our impulse to criticize ourselves. We are able to offer unconditional love to others despite their faults. And perhaps even more important, we are able to let ourselves off the hook and give ourselves the unconditional love that we always crave. As we learn to love ourselves, we let go of the negative energy that gets in the way of our joy. A balanced heart chakra enables us to receive and accept love when it is given to us. It enables us to feel connected to lovers, family, friends, and colleagues, banishing feelings of isolation and loneliness.

A Green Color Card Reading with Tina

The sweetest girl hesitantly walks up and requests a color card reading. She listens attentively as I explain that Tony&Tina Vibrational Remedies is a company dedicated to the idea that color, aroma, and thought can change and heal your life. As we begin, like most people, she is shocked to feel that strange sensation you get in your palm when you pick up the energy of the cards. She picks white and green. I explain that white, which represents the crown chakra, is where you get in touch with and reconnect to your spirituality. I tell her this is a time for her to focus on connecting her spiritual beliefs with her ethical code. I can tell she's confused. So I go on to tell her that white is cleansing to your energy system and she should look at whether there is a situation in her life that needs cleansing.

She begins to look emotional. I tell her about green and the heart chakra, that this is the place of unconditional love where you hold your grief and anger. The combination of white and green suggests there is something you need to let go of and cleanse. She bursts into tears as she tells me her husband of eight weeks has "changed his mind." She is utterly devastated and confused about the whole thing and what it says about her.

I immediately tell her she did nothing wrong and she needs to forgive herself. Women are quick to blame themselves when relationships fail and this is unnecessary. Balancing her white energy will help her connect with the Divine, which will give her comfort. It will also begin the process of cleansing the negativity she is holding in her heart chakra. Adding green energy will encourage her to love herself more and help her to let go of her grief.

When you are drawn to green you need to take stock, to see if you're holding on to grief and/or anger. When we hold on to negative emotions of hurt, anger, and resentment they take up space in this center and block the love you should be giving and receiving. You need to truly let these things go and allow space for positive new things to happen for you. Forgiveness is usually a big part of this process and forgiving ourselves is of utmost importance.

Many people pick green in our color card readings and when we tell them that the lesson here is forgiveness, the look on their faces is inevitably one of resistance. The lesson of forgiveness is one of the toughest. No one wants to forgive. Perhaps this is why it is the main teaching of the great masters of all religions. If we don't forgive, we continue to surrender power to the person who did us wrong. Some of us allow this drain to continue for many years, affecting our ability to love and be loved. It also affects our physical well-being. As the emotional origin of disease is understood, we begin to realize why bitterness, even as a response to an unforgivable wrong, is so detrimental to our health.

The law of karma is an incredibly accurate accounting system. No one gets away with anything. So release your desire for retribution and know that you don't forgive someone for their sake; you forgive them for yours.

This is a time in history of great global and personal change. Since it is the green energy that most aids personal transformation, we all need to "think green."

The Green Period of Our Relationship

For a year and a half after Tony and I broke up I was a totally green person. My heart chakra issues had taken over. Deep down, I knew our romantic relationship was over and we were stuck in many ways. We had to let each other go in order to begin growing again.

But first I needed to learn to love myself again; society had programmed me to believe I had failed and I needed the green energy to help me love myself more. The next step was to let go of grief and anger and forgive Tony. This was tough. You think "Hey, why am I doing all the work here?" And forgiveness really is work.

"If I have a hangover I always wear my green turtleneck. I like it because I've gotten compliments on it, and besides that it makes me feel safe. It's my safety shirt."
—Lisa

Lisa intuitively knows that green will fill her with love energy, and when we are filled with green love energy, we feel safe. Green also calms the nervous system, which is taxed if we've partied too hard the night before. Our suggestion to her would be to add a splash of blue and white because these colors are physically and mentally purifying.

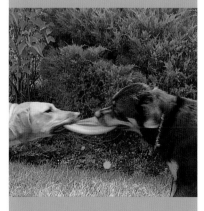

Green Issues

If you have too much green you may be:
- Too sensitive
- Demanding
- Judgmental
- Possessive
- Melodramatic
- Vulnerable to partaking in emotional blackmail

If you have too much green, you can balance by using green, followed by pink or soft reds.

If you have too little green you:
- Will have trouble letting go of grief and anger
- Don't forgive or trust people
- Feel sorry for yourself
- Are paranoid
- Are indecisive
- Feel unworthy of love
- Are frightened of rejection

If you have just enough green you are:
- Balanced
- Compassionate
- Empathetic
- One who sees the world with love
- In touch with your feelings
- Nurturing
- Friendly
- Forgiving

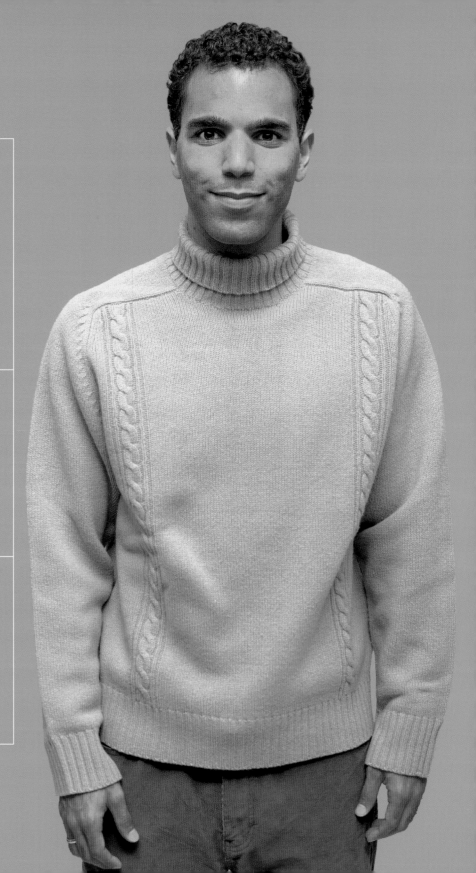

But there is no relief as profound as the relief you feel when you forgive. Forgiveness clears your energy system. You're not only letting go of negative energy, you're making new space available for joy and love. And let's face it folks, we can all use more love.

In order to begin a new relationship you need to make a complete separation from the last one. We helped the separation along through mutually disagreeable behavior. But we knew we still loved each other, and throughout the worst of the aftermath we still intended to be partners, just not in the man/woman kind of way. We're now able to open our hearts to each other with complete trust and unconditional love . . . well, at least when our egos are on holiday.

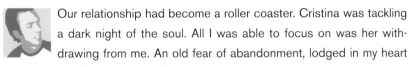 Our relationship had become a roller coaster. Cristina was tackling a dark night of the soul. All I was able to focus on was her withdrawing from me. An old fear of abandonment, lodged in my heart chakra as a child, resurfaced. Our needs were in opposition and we were just holding too much resentment and blame toward each other. Bless us. We needed a change, bad. The issues of the heart chakra are forgiveness and compassion, blame and grief. The last two we had in spades. We had become like a spiteful, nagging old couple from a sitcom, but it wasn't very funny.

We were both wondering how we could talk about color as a healing and transforming energy if we were manifesting our most unfavorable aspects. Then it dawned on me: when we are ready to deal with the lessons of the heart we are sent a test. The universe makes sure we have to dig deep and find it in our hearts to forgive.

Visualization

Sit for a few minutes and imagine your heart area glowing in your ideal green. See the glow spreading with every breath. You are letting go of all grief, anger, and pain. You are being suffused with pure love energy. This love energy is extending outward, as far outward as your mind will take you, into the infinite universe. Feel the love energy flowing out and feel the abundant love energy flowing in. Breathe it in.

GREEN FACTOIDS

Every culture and religion attributes positive qualities to green. Yet green, like yellow and red, has its share of negative associations, too. Throughout history, green has been the symbol of the soul's regeneration, but it has also signified moral degradation and madness. It is still associated with jealousy (hence "green with envy" and "the green-eyed monster").

The Druids considered green the color of learning.

In Christian symbolism green—being equidistant from the blue of heaven and the red of hell—is an intermediate and mediating color, the color of contemplation. Christ's cross, as a symbol of hope, is often portrayed as green as is the Holy Grail.

In Islam, green is the color of the Prophet Muhammad, believed to have been attended by angels in green turbans.

And in China, green jade has long been considered a lucky stone.

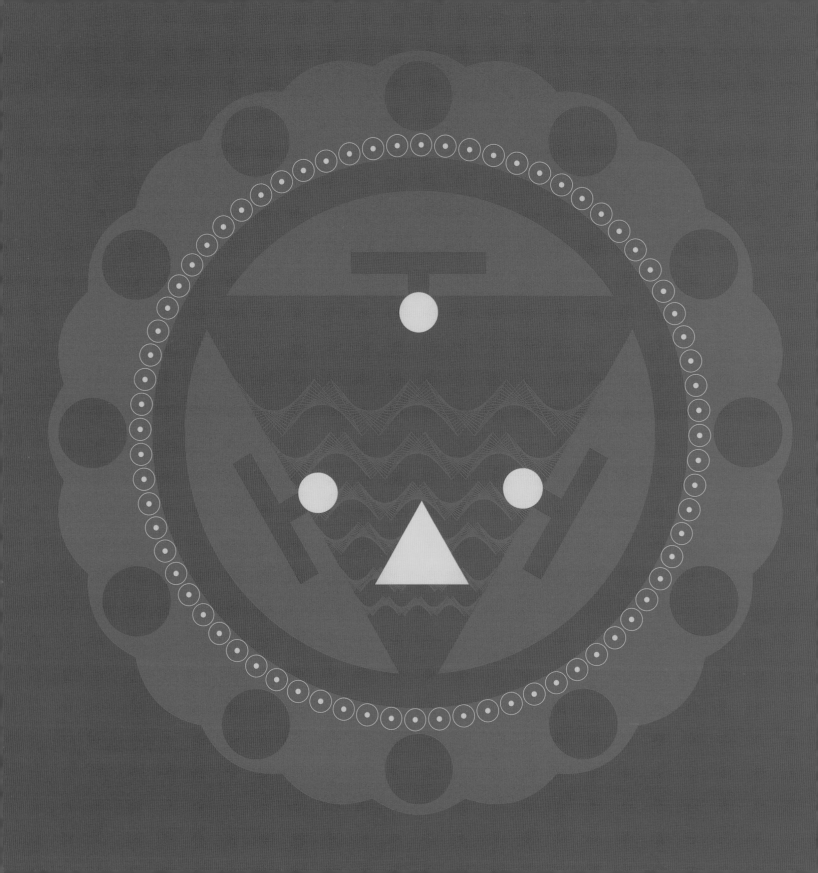

Blue: Communication

element: ether / planet: jupiter / signs: gemini and virgo / crystal: aquamarine / gemstone: sapphire / essential oil: eucalyptus / main life lesson: speaking your truth

The electromagnetic vibrations emitted by blue exactly match the frequency of the fifth chakra, which is located in the throat and related to the thyroid gland. This chakra is about self-expression, communication, knowledge, and wisdom. It is where we find our higher potential and manifest our dreams. **When this chakra is well-balanced, we express ourselves with truth and love.**

Ancient Hindu texts refer to the fifth chakra as the Vishuddha, or purification, chakra, where the divine nectar of immortality resides, in a secretion from a gland near the back of the throat. (This gland, the thyroid, can be stimulated through yogic practice. Master yogis credit their ability to live without food or water for long periods of time to its manipulation.)

The blue throat chakra is the center that asks if you are living according to your beliefs and ideals. Are you communicating effectively and honestly? Is there a situation in which you feel you are compromising yourself? Is there a person to whom you have something to say but you haven't said it? When you do these things, you metaphorically swallow your truth and this creates a blockage that usually manifests as depression or a physical problem in the throat.

"I have this light blue shirt I've started wearing lately. I was never really attracted to it before. I actually wore it my first day at my new job. I consider it my confidence shirt."

—Lisa

"Growing up on the ocean has created in me a natural attraction to watery shades of blue and green. They calm me. I am drawn to these colors as though they have mystical powers."

—Amber

This young woman's instincts are working perfectly not only because blue promotes confidence but because it also encourages effective communication, just what you need at a new job. This light shade of blue helps to relax her, which is also a plus during periods of change.

Blue energy encourages your true individuality and your ability to make decisions and stick to them. The blue center also strengthens your connection to divine intelligence. When you trust that everything happens for a reason, you can be assured that, as long as you are living truthfully, your decisions will lead you to exactly where you need to be.

As with yellow and orange, the blue throat chakra helps us to manifest greater abundance in our lives by giving us the strength of will and the enthusiasm to turn our dreams into realities.

A Blue Color Card Reading with Tina

The woman sat down in front of me, practically twitching. After she picked blue, the color she was also wearing, she told me her story. She had gotten a very good but high-pressure job five years ago with a company in severe financial difficulties. There were frequent layoffs and constant demands for her to increase the quarterly projections for her department. Morale was terrible, the atmosphere was oppressive, and she felt as if everyone was about to stab her in the back.

Some months after she took the job, she began to get sick. She was diagnosed with breast cancer and had a tumor removed, but more lumps appeared. After three years of this she was completely demoralized, her zest for life totally shot. She didn't confide to anyone at work about her health problems—neither her boss nor her colleagues—fearing she would be fired. She had managed to take very little time off after her surgeries for fear she would come back to "find someone else sitting in my desk." She had no friends at work and just tried to keep her head down. Absorbing the negativity of the company and withdrawing from her coworkers, she was in a terrible energy situation.

When I pointed out the obvious connection between her illnesses and her job, tears welled up. "You need to quit your job," I told her, and she seemed to come to life for the first time. "Oh, I *know* I have to quit," she said. I told her that the fact that she chose blue and was wearing blue showed that her intuition was working, that she had the confidence to make a change. She knew what she needed. She just needed to hear it spoken aloud.

The Blue Period of Our Relationship

It took separation to give us the space to start to really communicate again, and by using blue chakra energy things began to get very interesting between Tina and me. With our newfound compassion we stopped blaming each other and truly took equal responsibility for our breakup. This liberated us from the illusions we had created during our time together that made separation so painful. With the new energy from the throat chakra, we found the discipline, as individuals, to pull ourselves out of our respective slumps. We started to trust that there was a divine plan for us and we began to go with the flow.

After our breakup, after all the fighting and hating, we had to struggle to become separate individuals. Slowly we were able to really see each other and appreciate each other again. It took work to let go of our relationship and all our old patterns, but the value of our partnership was great enough, on a personal as well as a business level, that we were motivated to work through the problems. Blue color energy supported us.

After we broke up I was especially inexperienced at being alone. I had never lived on my own and had never lived my life answering only to myself. Blue energy encouraged me to develop my own truth and to be me, an individual willing to accept that everything that was happening to me should be happening. I began to gather the will to change the parts of myself I was unhappy about. I realized that if everything happens for a reason, then I might as well enjoy each step of the way while I'm working toward a true self I'm proud of.

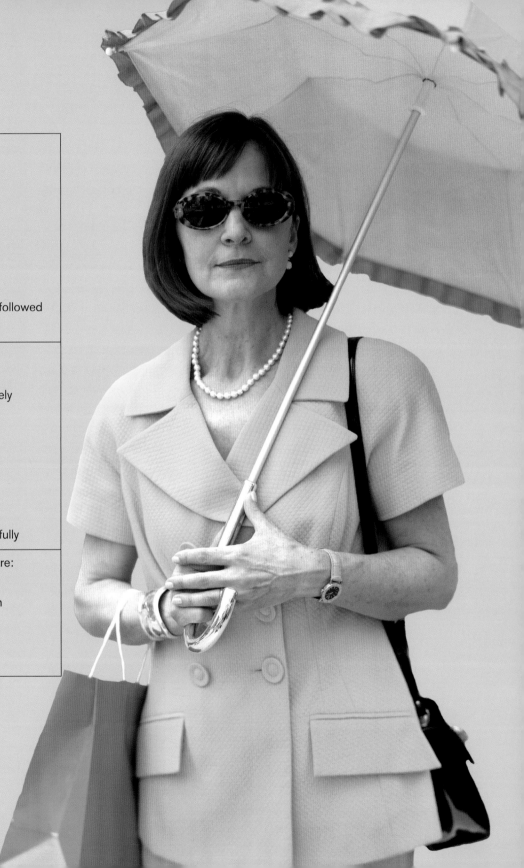

Blue Issues

If you have too much blue you:

- Will talk before you think
- May be anal
- Don't compromise
- Are arrogant
- Talk too much
- Are addictive
- Are self-righteous

You can balance by using orange followed by a small amount of blue.

If you have too little blue you are:

- Without self-control
- Unable to communicate effectively
- Likely to compromise too easily
- Timid
- Quiet
- Unreliable
- Inconsistent
- Devious
- Unable to express yourself truthfully

If you have just enough blue you are:

- Centered
- Able to live and speak your truth
- Able to live in the present
- A good speaker
- Artistic

Our environment can have a huge effect on us energetically, and it's easy to become mired in a situation that drains us. When we are aware of what is happening, we are able to use vibrational remedies to strengthen ourselves and our resistance to them.

A Follow-Up Blue Reading

Sometimes, in our readings, no particular issue comes up, but I find out, when I see this person again, that I have struck a chord after all. In one reading I talked to a girl about her blue chakra being the gates to her cosmic truth. She wrote me six months later and told me that when we met she had been addicted to crystal meth for four years, and that after our reading, she began to do the blue shower meditation I had shown her. On the sixth day, she said, she felt strong enough to go cold turkey. She said she had managed to stay free of drugs since then and was really getting into the I Ching.

Visualization

Breathe deeply for a few minutes. See yourself and the person or situation you want to work on surrounded by a blue light. Visualize yourself effectively communicating and taking action to positively resolve the issues. Know that your intentions come from love. Breathe this idea in.

Aqua

Aqua, a mixture of blue and green, is believed by color healers to be linked to a secondary chakra located between the heart and the throat. Associated with the thymus gland located in the chest, it has a strong effect on our immune system. Many healers believe that because we are polluting our planet and absorbing toxins into our bodies, this center will become more important in the years to come.

BLUE FACTOIDS

Most of the ancient gods, goddesses, and any force associated with the sky have been associated with the color blue. Native Americans, Buddhists, Hindus, and the Chinese all associate blue with the heavens. The Christians use the color to represent the Virgin Mary and the ancient Romans used it in association with Zeus and Venus. Vishnu, in ancient Indian myth, is colored blue, as is Krishna.

As is the case with other colors, however, blue can carry more than one meaning. Blue stones worn as amulets were used in many primitive civilizations to ward off the evil eye. In ancient China, demons and ghosts were depicted as blue-faced creatures, and more recently blue eyes, ribbons, and stripes were considered ugly and unlucky.

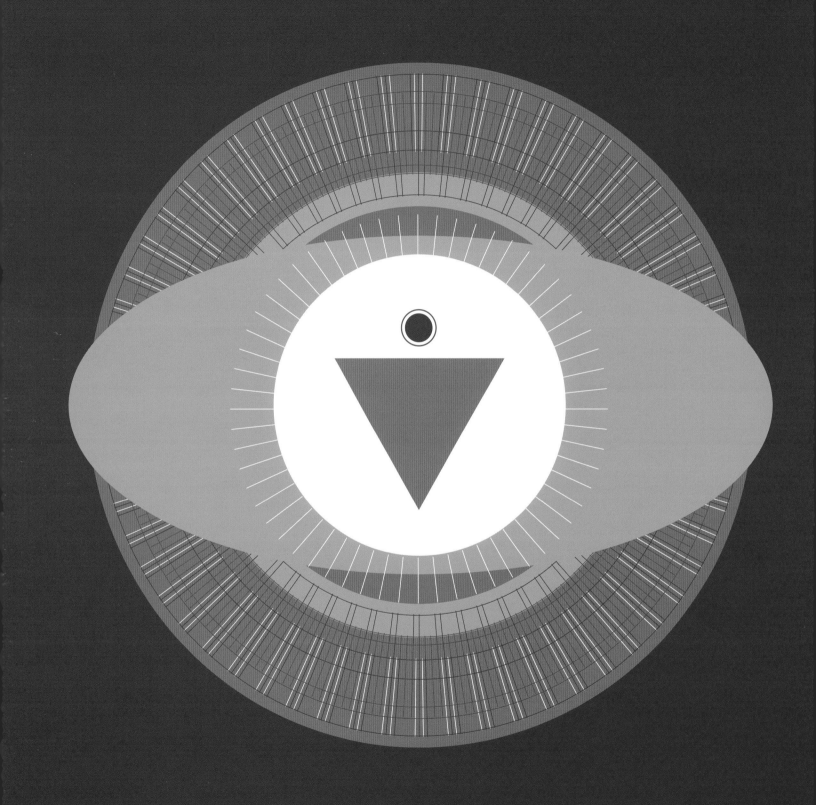

Violet: The Spirit

element: telepathic energy / sign: libra / crystal: amethyst / gemstone: purple ruby / essential oil: lavender / main life lessons: becoming conscious on all levels; perceiving the truth

The violet/purple frequency exactly matches the frequency of the sixth energy center. This chakra, located between the eyebrows, is linked to the pituitary gland. It emits the second highest frequency of the spectrum, lower only than white. Known as the third-eye chakra, this is the place where we connect to our spirit. It is the site of the knowledge and understanding that allows us to "see" intuitively. **This center, which regulates the energies between the physical and spiritual, enables us to activate our psychic powers and manifest our dreams.**

The violet chakra was known in ancient times as the "Ajna," or command, chakra—the place where we receive information from our source. The violet frequency helps to balance the left (rational) and right (intuitive) hemispheres of the brain. Some believe this is the center that can open us to our past-life experiences. This chakra opens the pathway between our conscious and our unconscious through intuition, wisdom, and detachment. It allows us to see the magic of our lives and how everything we experience has symbolic meaning and purpose.

When we have an overactive third-eye chakra we tend to be supersensi-

VIOLET FACTOIDS

Purple capes and robes have been worn for centuries by legendary rulers like the Caesars of ancient Rome. Peasants were forbidden to wear the color; to do so under Nero was punishable by death. The purple dye was made from the ink of a sea snail, and because it was difficult to come by, it became extremely valuable.

Purple vestments also played a part in Christian tradition. Worn by priests in their liturgical services, purple robes came to be associated with repentance, penance, expiation, and Christ's blood. Old representations of Christ's Passion show him wearing a violet mantle. Today, violet has become the color associated with advent and Easter.

Hopi Indians believe that over the next twelve years, our consciousness will evolve into the violet or third-eye chakra, ushering in a period of harmony, community consciousness, and peace.

tive and impatient, we worry a lot and go around with our head in the clouds. When the third-eye chakra is underactive we also worry and are prone to forgetfulness, may be superstitious, and have a fear of dying.

Right now, many of us are getting in touch with our higher selves and learning to consciously create our realities. Our psychic abilities are beginning to flourish. We've heard many other stories of intuitive events—how people know who's on the phone before they pick it up, have prophetic dreams, or think of someone and run into them as they turn the corner. More and more of us are tapped in. Third-eye consciousness is on the horizon!

 My father actually had a purple experience at my grandmother's funeral. He was hugging his wife, his eyes were shut, and suddenly, illuminated purple flooded across his mind's eye. He said in that moment, he vividly felt her presence.

When you are drawn to violet, it is time for you to connect with your spirit, reflect on your life fearlessly, and assess whether your opinions are outdated. This center allows you to detach and objectively look at the people and situations in your life, to feel your inner power and connect with your higher self.

A Violet Color Card Reading with Tony

A woman I gave a reading to picked violet. When I started to explain the realms of the spiritual body and our yearning for deeper levels of truth and understanding, she stopped me abruptly and told me that the worst thing that could happen to someone had happened to her. She told me that she had lost her husband and her two children in Flight 800, which went down over Scotland, and that she could not see the point in living any longer. Such extreme grief would threaten to blow the circuits of the heart if it were not for the intervention of the violet or third-eye energy. The third eye is the chakra that constantly guides us to reevaluate what we feel to be the truth. Here, in this energy center, we have the potential for merging our powers of reason with divine wisdom. The Hindus say that an open third eye allows us to see the illusions of this physical world and gives us a view into our past lives. Violet is also said

Us

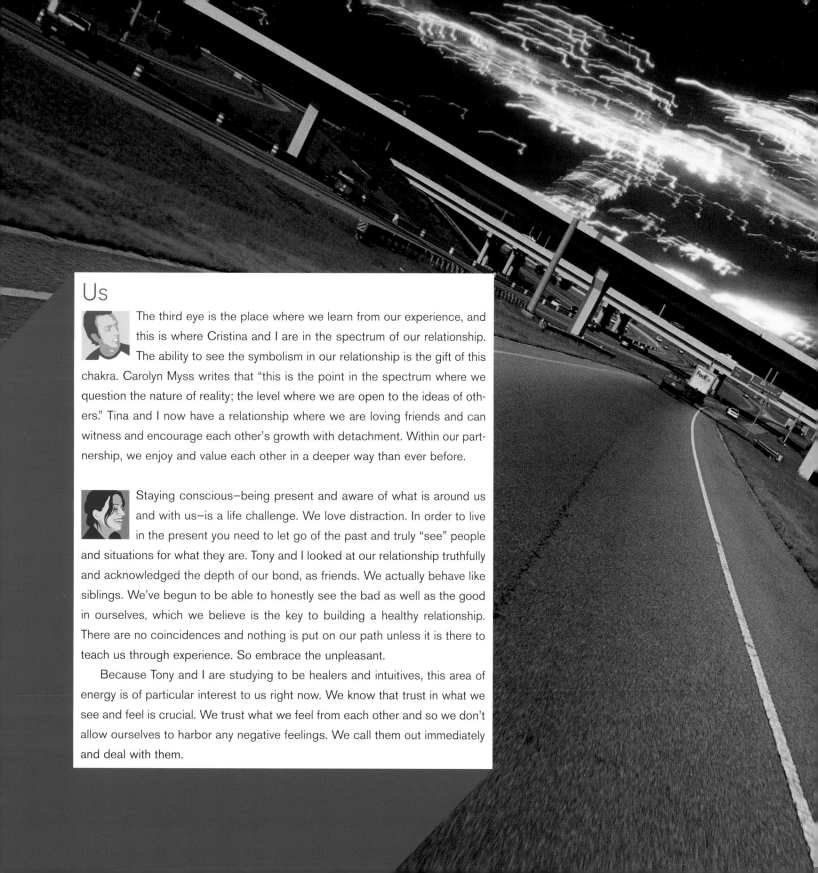

The third eye is the place where we learn from our experience, and this is where Cristina and I are in the spectrum of our relationship. The ability to see the symbolism in our relationship is the gift of this chakra. Carolyn Myss writes that "this is the point in the spectrum where we question the nature of reality; the level where we are open to the ideas of others." Tina and I now have a relationship where we are loving friends and can witness and encourage each other's growth with detachment. Within our partnership, we enjoy and value each other in a deeper way than ever before.

Staying conscious—being present and aware of what is around us and with us—is a life challenge. We love distraction. In order to live in the present you need to let go of the past and truly "see" people and situations for what they are. Tony and I looked at our relationship truthfully and acknowledged the depth of our bond, as friends. We actually behave like siblings. We've begun to be able to honestly see the bad as well as the good in ourselves, which we believe is the key to building a healthy relationship. There are no coincidences and nothing is put on our path unless it is there to teach us through experience. So embrace the unpleasant.

Because Tony and I are studying to be healers and intuitives, this area of energy is of particular interest to us right now. We know that trust in what we see and feel is crucial. We trust what we feel from each other and so we don't allow ourselves to harbor any negative feelings. We call them out immediately and deal with them.

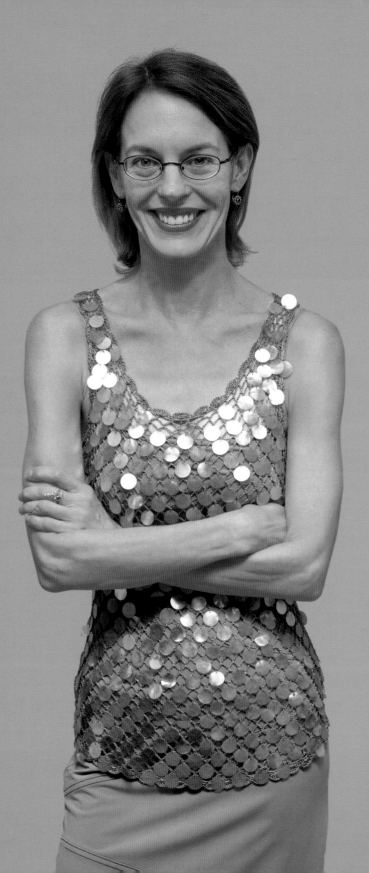

Violet Issues

If you have too much violet you may be:
- Going around with your head in the clouds
- Told you have a big ego
- Manipulative
- Authoritarian
- A religious fanatic

You can balance by adding yellow followed by a small amount of violet.

If you have too little violet you are:
- Oblivious to the messages that life shows you on a daily basis
- Unable to see things objectively
- Not assertive
- Undisciplined
- Highly sensitive
- Afraid of success

If you have just enough violet you are:
- Charismatic
- Connected to spirit
- Connected to the infinite wisdom
- Connected to cosmic consciousness
- Not attracted to material things
- Unafraid of death

to carry you to loved ones who have died and are sending you love from the other side.

As I told her all this, she listened intently, as though she was hearing a very important message from far away. I told her that experiencing loss of this magnitude is an indication of her role in our evolution into cosmic truth, that through the enduring teachings of reincarnation, we know that we travel from physical life to physical life in soul groups. A parent in this life may have played the role of a child in a past life. A lover in this life may have been a parent in the last. And so the loss of loved ones in this life is, in the truth of the violet chakra, but a moment's separation.

With the trust and wisdom of the third eye, we know that there is no separation even in death. With that knowledge, we must let go and move on.

Visualization

Sit in a quiet room, if possible, and do a few minutes of deep breathing. See your third eye glowing with violet light and connecting you to your spirit. You are calm and open to all information. You can see truth without making judgments. You can see people and situations as they really are, without fear or desire. You are allowing your intuitive wisdom to send messages to your conscious mind. You are open to everything you receive without judgments. Breathe it in.

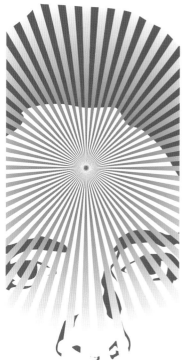

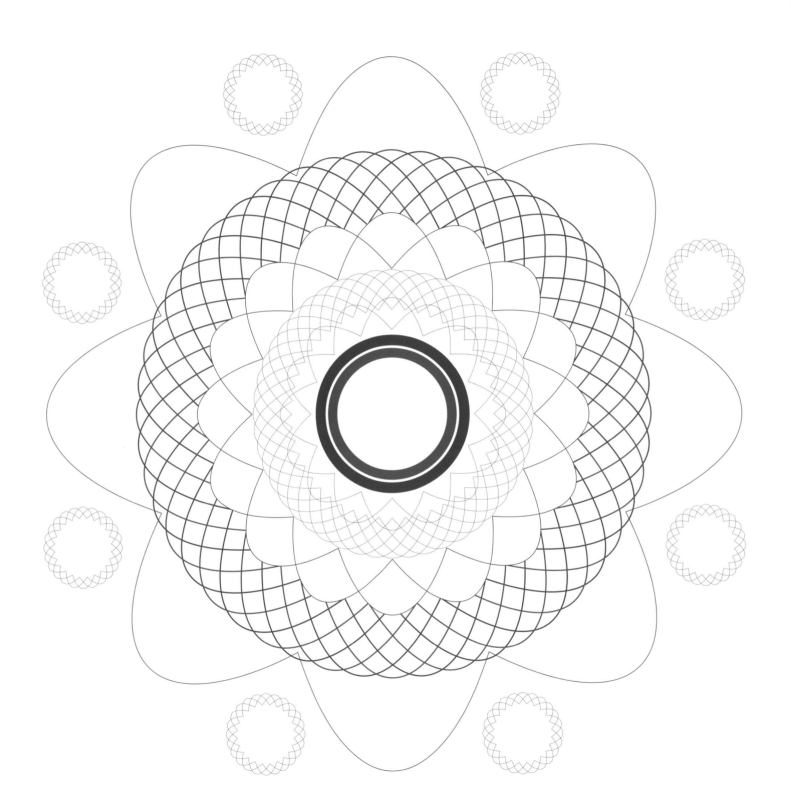

White: The Divine

element: cosmic energy / planet: moon / sign: cancer /
crystal: clear quartz / gemstone: diamond / essential oil:
jasmine / main life lesson: surrender to higher will

The electromagnetic frequency of white exactly matches the frequency of the
seventh energy center, or the crown chakra, located at the top of the head.
When this chakra is open, we experience oneness with the universe. The white
chakra is where our spiritual life is centered and where we achieve unity with
our source. This center is also associated with the pineal gland and is believed
to strongly affect the aging process.

In Hindu texts, this chakra is known as the *saharara* chakra, or the thou-
sand-petaled lotus. And since the number one thousand represents infinity,
this center connects us to our infinite source. Vedic texts associate white light
with Nirvana, the ultimate state of being. They explain that we—like the rainbow—are made of a white light whose origin is divine. In the Christian tradition,
white is also associated with God and the divine spirit.

The white energy center is responsible for inspiration and our connection
to the cosmos. **When our crown chakra is balanced, we experience a sense of oneness with the infinite and an understanding of our constantly unfolding spiritual nature.** This center allows
us to experience our connection to all sentient beings, so we become com-

WHITE FACTOIDS

White has been connected to spirit and purity by many cultures over thousands of years. The Hindus associated white with self-illumination, the Christians with purity, sainthood, and the Holy Spirit. In ancient times white animals were sacrificed to heavenly deities. In ancient Greece and Rome as well as the Orient, white was associated with mourning since it was believed that the dead were being reborn into a new pure state of being. By the same token, the white wedding dress also symbolizes not only a virginal state but the bride leaving the old behind and moving into the new.

In many cultures white garments (or those that were not dyed) were used as priestly vestments. Pythagoras recommended that singers of sacred hymns wear white and newly baptized Christians wore white robes.

In Chinese symbolic tradition, white is the color of virginity and purity but also of age, autumn, the West, and misfortune.

passionate and helpful to others. When our crown chakra is out of balance we lack inspiration and feel confused, depressed, and alienated. We become mired in our own problems and reluctant to reach out to those in need.

White is particularly effective getting rid of negativity. Because white has such a strong cleansing vibration, it is one of the best colors to use as you begin to incorporate color remedies into your daily life.

When you are drawn to white, you need to find out which aspect of your life needs cleansing. It could be a situation you find yourself in, or it could be a condition within. An attraction to white energy can mean it is time for you to reconnect with your source, your spirituality. Look at your life. Are you living it in accordance with your spiritual beliefs? Do you ask for more than you give? Are you tolerant of the spiritual beliefs of others? Have you cleared out any negative or blocked energy that might be hampering your connection to spirit? Are you meditating? The white energy allows you to go into your quiet space and see the glory of you and your relationship with the universe.

A White Color Card Reading

An older woman sat with me and picked white. We talked about how, when you are attracted to this energy, you need to reconnect with your spirit and cleanse. I also told her that needing white can be associated with skeletal and immune problems. She looked very surprised. She did have an autoimmune disorder, she said, and had been told she had less than two years to live. Receiving this news about her own mortality had been shattering to her, but now, three or four months had passed and she felt relief. "I'm now living in the present in a way that I never could before," she told me. At this point it was her family and the other people who loved her who were having the hardest time.

Because white energy is about spirit and being present, it made complete sense that she had chosen the white color card. Even with her dire prospects, this woman seemed very calm and serene. She told me she had been attracted to the white energy for some time now. She realized she'd been wearing it a lot and had been buying white things for the house. After our reading, she decided to incorporate a white color shower into her daily meditation ritual.

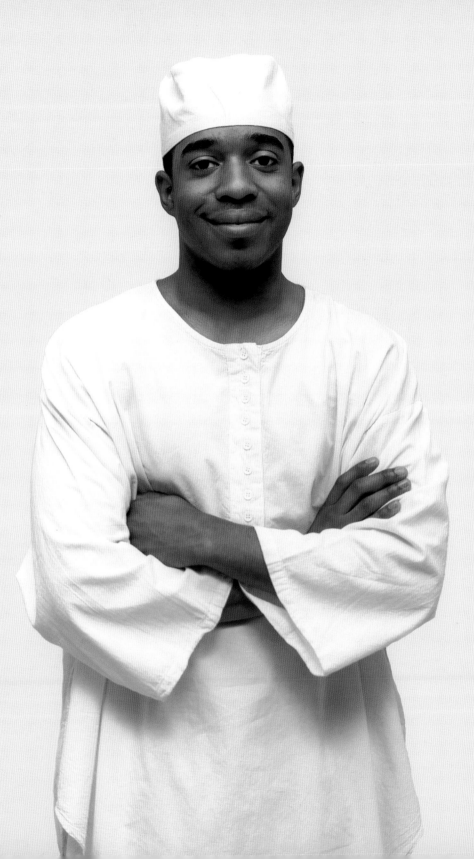

White Issues

If you have too much white you:
- May become easily frustrated
- Don't reach your full potential
- Are depressed
- Are destructive

You can balance by adding red followed by a small amount of white.

If you have too little white you:
- May live in conflict to your spiritual beliefs
- Are depressed
- Are indecisive

If you have just enough white you are:
- Open to the divine
- Able to live life in accordance with your spiritual beliefs
- Cleansed of all negativity and blocks
- Able to transcend our materialistic reality

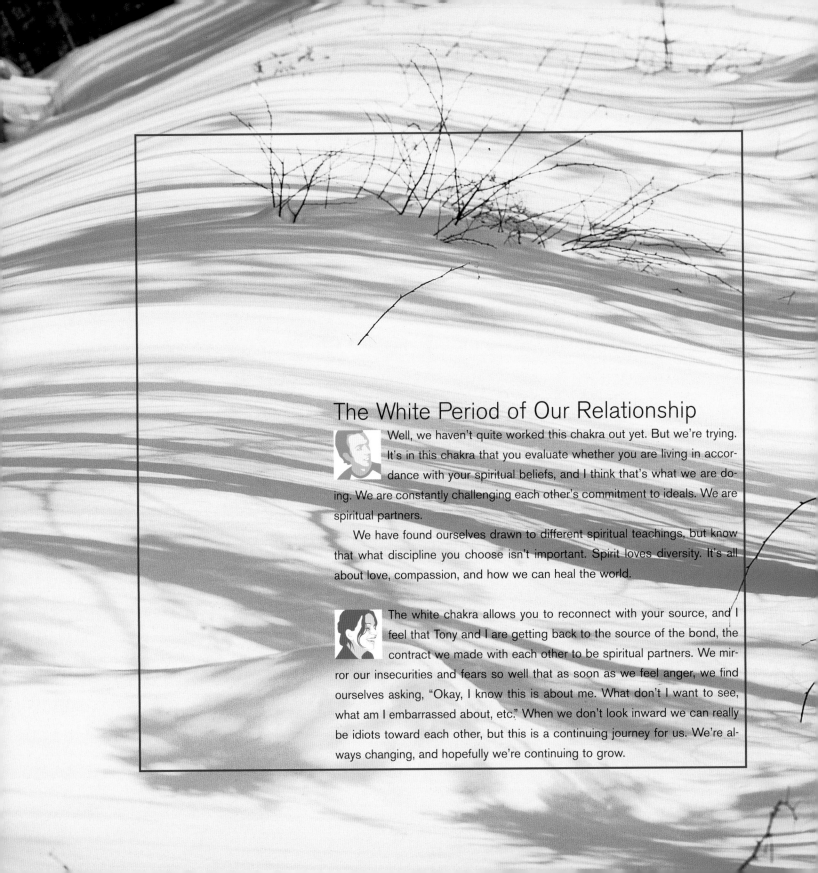

The White Period of Our Relationship

Well, we haven't quite worked this chakra out yet. But we're trying. It's in this chakra that you evaluate whether you are living in accordance with your spiritual beliefs, and I think that's what we are doing. We are constantly challenging each other's commitment to ideals. We are spiritual partners.

We have found ourselves drawn to different spiritual teachings, but know that what discipline you choose isn't important. Spirit loves diversity. It's all about love, compassion, and how we can heal the world.

The white chakra allows you to reconnect with your source, and I feel that Tony and I are getting back to the source of the bond, the contract we made with each other to be spiritual partners. We mirror our insecurities and fears so well that as soon as we feel anger, we find ourselves asking, "Okay, I know this is about me. What don't I want to see, what am I embarrassed about, etc." When we don't look inward we can really be idiots toward each other, but this is a continuing journey for us. We're always changing, and hopefully we're continuing to grow.

Other Important Chakras

We have focused on the body's seven primary energy centers, but it is important to note that we also have three external chakras. There is some disagreement among healers and intuitives as to how these energy centers relate to the other chakras, there is no disagreement about their characteristics.

The SILVER, or eighth, chakra is located below our feet and is described in Eastern philosophies as female energy. This energy is a centripetal force that originates in the earth, is drawn in through the feet and upward, spiraling around the uterus, breasts, and tonsils.

The GOLD, or ninth, chakra is described as male energy. Located above our heads, it moves down through the throat, heart, solar plexus, and genitals. Both men and women are connected to the gold and silver chakras, but silver is stronger in women and gold is stronger in men.

The third external chakra is the BLACK, or twelfth, chakra, and it is located below the silver. Its function is to push us forward. It is interesting to note that Kali, the Hindu goddess of destruction and rebirth, is depicted as black. And throughout history, black has carried negative connotations such as black magic and black mood, perhaps because we all have an inherent fear of change. In any case, we need to constantly move forward, and black color energy assists us in displacing stale energy.

The transmitter chakras, considered the tenth and eleventh chakras, are TRANSPARENT and are located in the palm of each hand. They are of special importance because they can be effectively used in transmitting energy. As anyone involved in body work knows, they are our healing tools. The dominant hand is usually the transmitter and the other hand the receiver. Every joint is a secondary chakra and so the many joints in the fingers and wrists add to the power of energy transmitted and received through the hands.

In this light, a handshake becomes a whole new story. When we shake hands we are actually exchanging energy with another person, giving us a sense of their personality and their physical state. (See page 84 for using the hands to positively manipulate energy through color and intention.)

MALE/FEMALE ENERGY

An imbalance between our male and female energies is the source of many woes. We learned this exercise from the teacher and writer Alihandra in her book *Healing with the Rainbow Ray.* She explains that when our male and female selves aren't talking, our thoughts and actions are out of sync. If you feel you have many ideas that you can never seem to bring to fruition, your male energy isn't supporting your female energy. If you find yourself treating other people with harsh disregard, your female energy isn't supporting your male energy. To balance, try this exercise once each week:

1. Picture a gold ray that is male energy showering down through your head, down to your heart chakra, turning clockwise.

2. Then picture a silver ray that is female energy moving up through your feet to your heart chakra and turning counterclockwise.

3. See them begin to merge together.

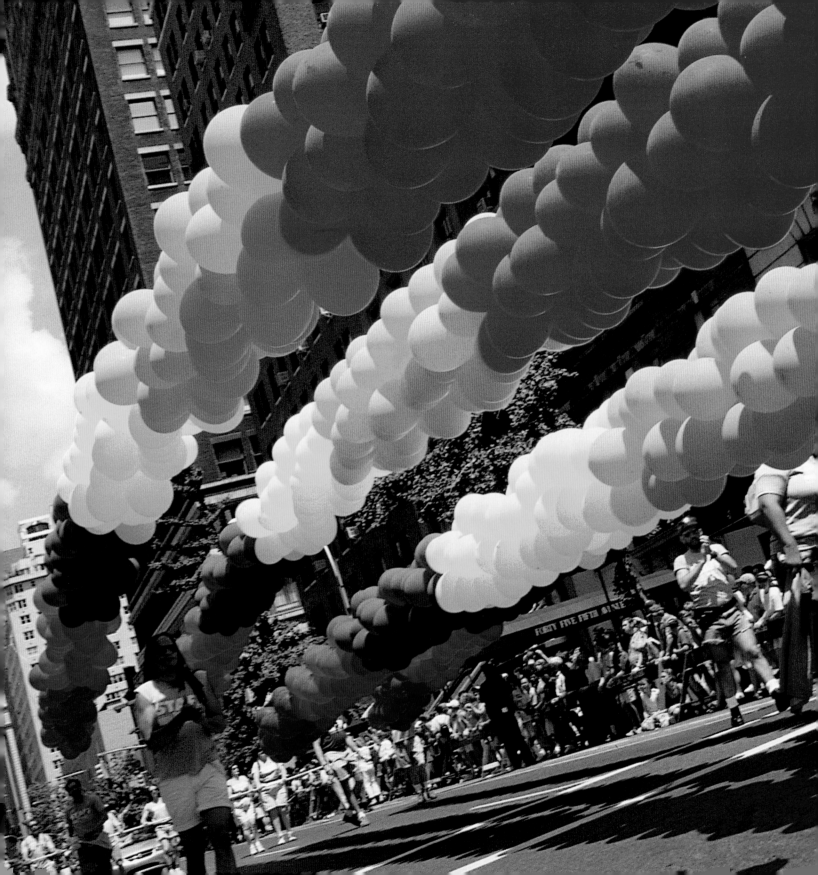

Part II
Feeding Yourself Color Energy

Exercises to Boost Your Color Energy

To determine which color or colors will be most effective in balancing your energy centers, do a color card reading or check with a pendulum (see pages 24 and 27). Once you've done this, you can actually feed yourself color energy using any of these exercises. Read through all of them to find those that appeal to you the most and then try them to see which ones are most effective. Most are very easy to do, and if you practice them day after day, you will find yourself increasingly sensitive to their effects. You can also refer to the Healing Chart (page 117) for colors to use in healing physical conditions.

Before you begin any color energy exercise, take a few minutes to prepare yourself with deep rhythmic breathing (page 116). This will help your body receive the color energies.

The Color Shower

The color shower is extremely effective in balancing your chakras. For instance, if you're feeling anxious, a blue color shower will help you calm down.

1. Decide which color you need.

2. Prepare yourself with a few minutes of deep breathing.

3. Picture the most perfect shade of your color. See it in your mind's eye showering down from the universe into the crown of your head, down through your body, down through each arm, down each leg, and out through your feet.

4. The color energy is smart energy. It will go where it is needed and encourage any blocks or negativity to drain away. It feels refreshing.

The breathing should take about fifteen seconds and the visualization about a minute. Longer is always better. This shouldn't be a three-second experience unless you are pressed for time and need just a quick burst of energy.

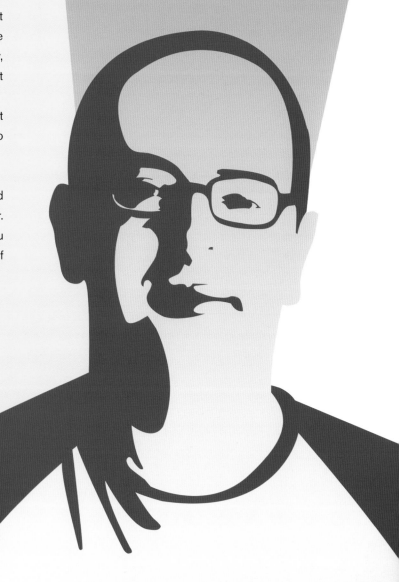

The White Bubble Technique

White is a protective energy. This technique is excellent for those times when you feel negative vibrations from people or when you're in a difficult or even threatening situation.

 The first time I visualized a white bubble was at a camp when I was a child. I was scared of things that went bump in the night so I imagined I was surrounded by this illuminated white bubble and suddenly I felt safe. At age ten I certainly didn't know from color therapy—this is a good example of our instincts leading us to exactly what we need.

1. Assuming you're not in immediate danger, prepare yourself with deep breathing.

2. Visualize yourself completely surrounded by a big white energy bubble that extends six to twelve inches away from your body. Feel yourself being cleansed of negative energy and protected from any negative energy around you.

3. You can also visualize the bubble around another person, place, or situation. When I feel anxious on a plane, which is often, I visualize a white bubble surrounding the entire thing. It stays there for the duration of the flight and protects all the other planes flying that day as well.

Shakti Gawain describes a technique where you visualize exactly what you want and send it off into the universe in a pink bubble. This technique worked for us; in fact we credit it with launching our company.

Breathing in Color

This technique is especially useful for healing physical conditions. Refer to the Healing Chart (page 117) to identify the color(s) that can help your condition. For example, pink and light blue breath is beneficial for skin. Red breath helps with colds and sinus conditions. Blue breath eases respiratory problems and is generally good for children.

1. If possible, and assuming you don't live in a highly polluted area, do this exercise outdoors or sit by an open window.

2. Prepare yourself with deep breathing.

3. Imagine the color you want to take in. Breathe it in as colored light. Your thoughts will change the energy of the air you are breathing in.

Taking a Color Sunbath

A simple and pleasurable way to take in color energy is through colored glass. You can easily create colored glass by buying sheets of colored cellophane at an art supply store. Sheets thirty-six inches square are ideal, but smaller is fine, too. This exercise needs to be done on a sunny day.

1. Decide which color you need to balance.

2. Tape your sheet of colored cellophane to the lower half of a sunny window.

3. Sit in front of the window so that the sun is streaming through the cellophane onto your body. Breathe deeply for ten minutes or so.

This technique has been used by many color therapists to heal physical conditions.

Spinning the Chakras

With this exercise you can balance all your chakras or any one of them individually. Before you begin, test all your chakras with a pendulum. This should indicate that they're all spinning strongly in a clockwise direction.

1. Prepare yourself with deep rhythmic breathing.

2. Lie down and hold a pendulum above your body. Check one chakra at a time, beginning with the red chakra.

3. If you find that the pendulum is not spinning clockwise, just keep holding it steady. It will stop and slowly reverse direction.

4. Once your chakras are all spinning clockwise, set the pendulum aside.

5. Visualize the color of the chakra you want to work on.

6. Imagine the chakra spinning three times to the right and then three to the left.

7. To rebalance all of your chakras, start with red and work your way up through orange, yellow, green, blue, violet, and white. You will not only be balancing your chakras but your male and female energy as well.

"It seems clear that light is the most important environmental input after food in controlling bodily function."
—Richard T. Wurtman, nutritionist

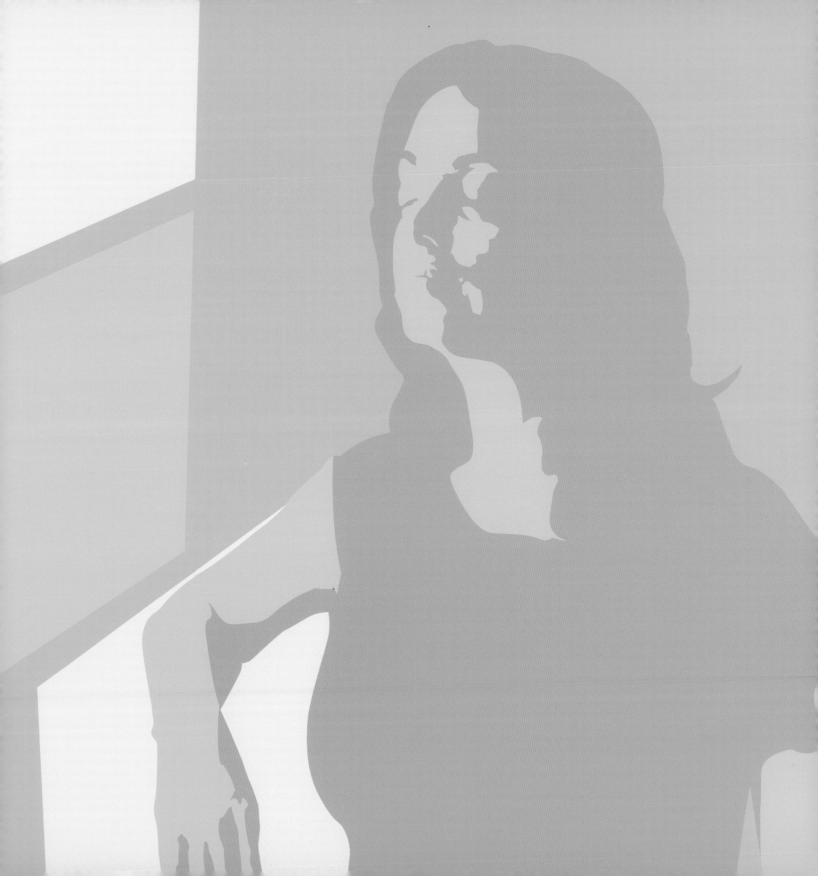

Colored Fabric Swatches

A simple way to balance the chakras after a stressful day is to place a swatch of colored cotton cloth over the chakra in need of balancing. You can buy squares of colored cotton in any fabric store.

1. Prepare yourself with a few minutes of deep breathing.

2. Lie down and place the swatch over the chakra you are working on, or you can place a swatch over each of the seven chakras if you wish to balance them all.

3. Breathe deeply into the areas covered with swatches. Mentally affirm to yourself that you are balancing your energy system. Do this for five minutes, but if one minute is all you can muster, we'll take it.

Solarizing Water

The benefits of drinking water can be maximized by creating solarized water with one of the seven color frequencies. We first read about this in Theo Gimbel's *Healing with Color and Light*.

1. Decide which chakra you want to balance and choose your color accordingly.

2. Take a transparent glass or transparent plastic container of the color you require.

3. Fill the glass with water and place it in the sun for several hours, longer if the day is cloudy.

4. After several hours in the sun, the water will be infused with the vibrations of the color. Sip it slowly and reap the benefits.

5. Keep the water in the refrigerator. Do not keep the water from the warm end of the spectrum more than a few days. The cool colored water can be kept a few days longer.

You can vary this exercise by using seven different glasses, one for each of the different chakra colors, and solarizing them all at once. When we tried this, we found that the water from each glass had a distinctly different taste.

You can also wrap a clear glass or jar with transparent fabric the color of the chakra you wish to work on. Silk is ideal. The sun will penetrate the fabric and solarize the water.

A healer once gave me yellow water to drink after determining that I allowed myself to be affected too much by the energy of other people, thus draining my solar plexus. I drank the water for four days and put a few drops directly on my third chakra center. I really felt a difference.

Color Meditation

Color meditation is a particularly easy and effective exercise. Here are the steps:

1. To determine a color for your meditation, visualize each of the chakra colors in turn. One or two of them will resonate. Trust your inner wisdom to guide you as to which ones to use. Breathe.

2. With each inhalation, imagine the color surrounding you and with each exhalation imagine it showering down into the top of your head, flowing through your body, and washing out through your feet. Your thought, your most powerful vibrational remedy, will introduce that particular color frequency into your body. You will be reaping the therapeutic benefits by changing the frequency of the air you are breathing.

3. Allow the color to take form and dance within your mind's eye. The experience is different for everyone, so see it as you see it, feel it as you feel it.

4. You can finish your meditation with another color if you like. Meditate on white to cleanse negativity and your overall system, green to heal internal organs and hurt emotions, pink to cleanse your aura, or blue to calm you.

We suggest doing the color meditation in the morning and before bed for five to fifteen minutes.

Projecting Color

Projecting color through your hand is a technique primarily used for healing specific areas of the body. The instructions below are for healing another person, but you can also use this exercise on yourself. Projecting color is a remarkable tool, and when you become proficient with it, you can even branch out into long-distance healing. Before you begin to exchange energy with someone else, be sure to ground and balance yourself with the Four Essentials for Healing (page 118).

1. Determine which color your friend needs.
2. Ask permission from your friend to help him or her heal.
3. Ask your friend to spend a few minutes doing deep rhythmic breathing.

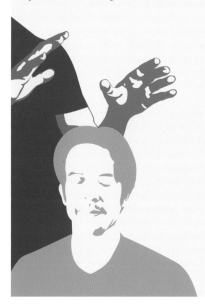

4. Extend your dominant hand out in front of you.
5. Imagine the crown at the top of your head opening up to the universe. Repeat to yourself: "I am an open channel to the love and light of the universe."
6. Imagine the most perfect shade of the color you require. Ask your friend to visualize it, too.
7. Ask that the color be channeled in through your head and out through your hand.
8. Place your hand over the area of your friend's body that needs help.
9. Visualize this color energy flowing into your friend's body, alleviating illness and pain.

A young friend who tried this said, matter-of-factly, "I pictured my head opening up and these colors rushing in, down my arm, and into your body. It's really cool."

We agree, very cool.

 I used this technique with a friend who had an impossible case of the hiccups. I knew that blue, being an anti-inflammatory, would help calm her spasms. We closed our eyes and I put one hand over her upper chest. Breathing deeply, I imagined blue coming out of my hand and entering her. Within a few seconds my hand became so hot it felt like there was a ball of energy between us. She felt it, too. About thirty seconds later, we opened our eyes and her hiccups were gone.

Whatever works, you know.

Making Art

Painting is a great way to feed yourself color energy and to work through and/or discover emotional blockages. We all feel the impulse to create—if we could stop reminding ourselves of our limitations long enough and just do it. My mum used to take me to art galleries when I was quite young, and something she once said made me aware for the first time of what I wanted to do with my life. We were at a pop art show, when she looked at me with resignation and said, "Artists are allowed to do anything these days." Well, that seemed like the job for me.

Painting has led me through each stage in my personal evolution. Every time I find myself at a dead end, the act of painting has helped me to work through my difficulties with faith. When, halfway through a painting, I see that it is not turning out as I had hoped, I start to feel lost. But I work on, allowing the harmonics of one color to suggest its neighbor, and the flow of one shape to force another shape. The whole process is a metaphor for all aspects of my life.

The more I can silence my chattering mind and just allow the painting to unfold, the more the honesty of the work comes through.

Except for my most rambunctious moments, years ago, when I was known to grab spray paint and go at the walls, I had been painting in drawing books. So when I moved into a bigger apartment, I decided it was time to start buying canvas. I remember feeling a buzz the Saturday I woke up early to

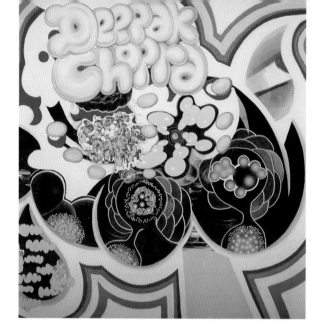

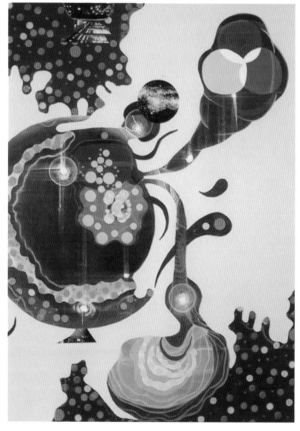

go down to Pearl Paint, the art supply store in China-town. I put on my Walkman and, listening to Veruca Salt and Hole, I felt vibed. I had never been in Pearls before and was excited by how big it is. I bought lots of extra things—like molding mud—in case I possibly wanted the three-dimensional look. When I finally got to the base-ment, where they keep the canvas, my hands were full, but that didn't stop me from buying three of the biggest canvases I could find, each measuring at least four by six feet.

On the subway ride home, I was holding back big smiles because I noticed that people were looking at me differently. They looked curious, probably wondering whether I was any good and whether they should re-member me. I liked the feeling of people thinking I was an artist, and it made me realize how awesome people think artists are, how easily you can be perceived as one, and how, when you do it, good or bad, you *are* one.

Society has conditioned us to think that we must be trained or have a natural talent to partake in making art. Not so. I am a very emotional untrained painter, but it wasn't until I met Tony that I began to trust what I was doing. I would beg him to teach me figurative tech-niques, but he refused. The most important thing he taught me was that style comes out of imperfection and the struggle to get an image down. After a while I came to see his point.

So, for all of you who swear you don't have an artis-tic side, plunging in and just doing is a great way to prove yourself wrong. As you buy your materials, re-member that the most important thing on your list is your intention to let go of your preconceptions about art.

Although what I've made is an indistinct, abstract shape, when I look at it I usually end up feeling relief be-cause I've downloaded onto the paper some stale or negative energy. Sometimes even just making a line or two makes me feel better.

Of course, painting doesn't always have to be the purging of negativity. It can be a celebration of spirit, like this one. Experience the joy of what it's like to just feel present.

Let the drawing or painting take its own shape. Al-low the awkwardness. Life is full of ups and downs, happiness, and pain, so not all expressions are going to be pleasing. If they are honest, they become beautiful.

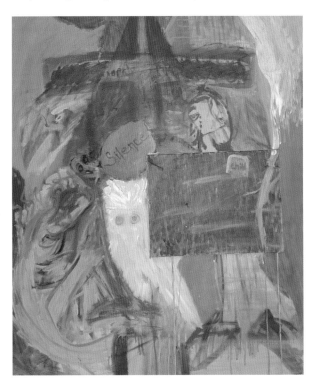

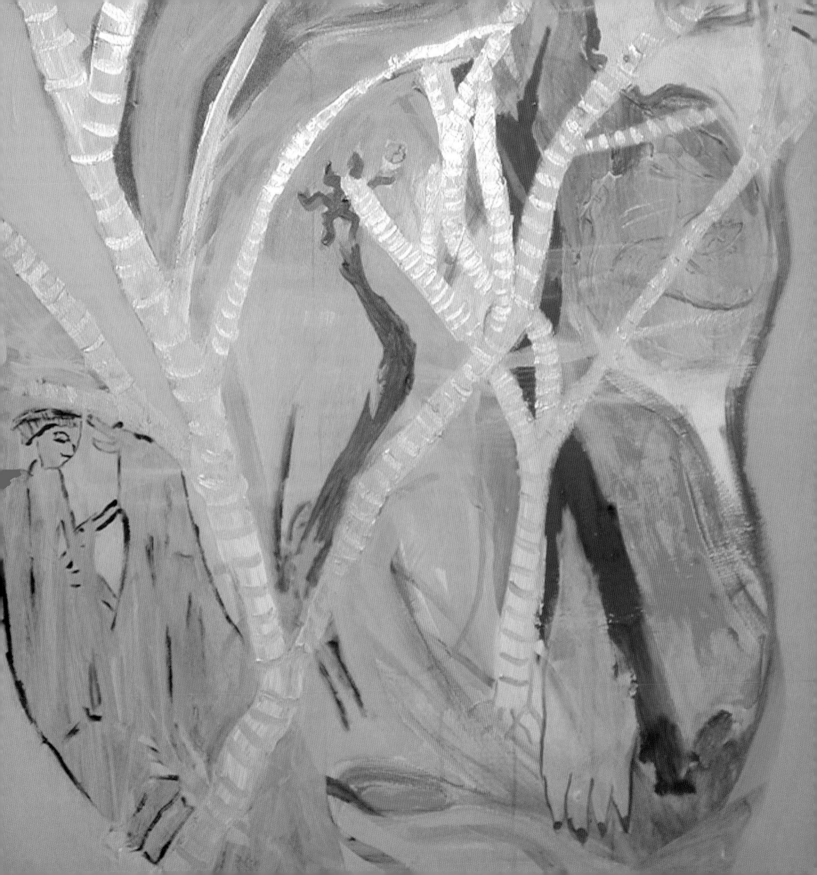

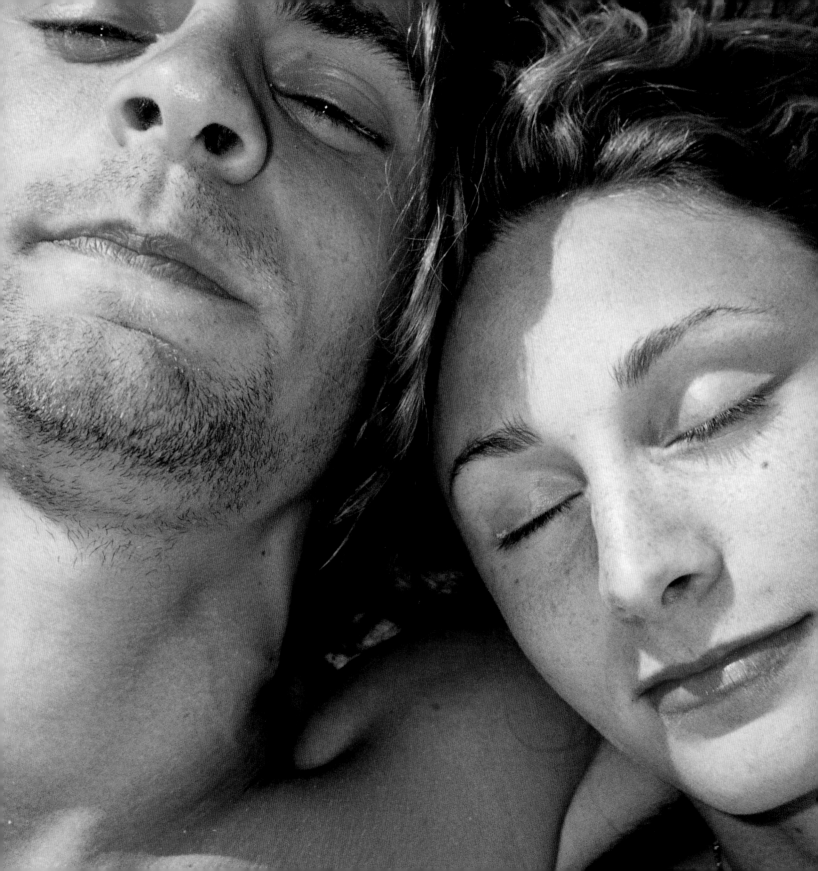

Part III
Apply Liberally—Practical Applications

The Colors of Love

Just as the heart is the engine of our physical body, so love is our fuel. As the Beatles put it, "All you need is love." Love energy—green chakra energy—is what many of us spend an enormous amount of our time thinking about and acting upon. **When we love, we are in sync with our true nature and with the flow of the universe; we are happy; we let go of fear.** Fear is an illusion created by our ego mind; it causes us to read into situations and make problems where there are none. Love is the only truth, the only reality. Love is a panacea, an elixir that allows us to live in harmony with ourselves and our world. Love is the presence of the Divine in us. To love unconditionally is our greatest life lesson; it is the reason we are here.

Loving Yourself

Love manifests in many different ways—love for family, for friends, for a partner, for a place or an idea. But love for yourself is primary. We need to truly love who we are, not who we were or want someday to be but who we are, just as we are. Instead of comparing ourselves with everyone around us, we need to accept that we are all unique and be glad to be ourselves, alive, living our lives with the opportunity to learn and change.

Our need for love is so huge. Most people who are chronically unhappy develop negative emotional patterns and feel rejected, and believe in some way they don't deserve love. But when our sense of self is strong, we can catch ourselves before we succumb to these feelings. We have the courage to understand that we are in no way diminished just because someone chooses not to be with us. Maybe rejection was necessary to give us time for self-reflection. Maybe a relationship needed to be dissolved so that a better one could begin. Breakups give us new lives and that can be very exciting if we let go of our fear of being alone.

It is in our nature to form intimate relationships. We need positive, intimate contact with others to keep our energy flowing. We will always find people who can love us and whom we can love, and we never need to be alone for long unless that is the path we choose. We cannot depend on others to infuse us with love. When we love ourselves, treat ourselves with the kindness and the unconditional acceptance that we seek from others, then we will attract the love we want.

To be in love–to merge and lose yourself with another–is the idealistic dream. But the realization of this dream usually means that either one or both partner sustains a terrible loss of individual power, creating a fundamental energy imbalance. To lose yourself in your own self-love is an entirely different matter, but it can give the same beautiful high.

It's very empowering to know you can fill yourself with the positive energy a lover would have provided.

Having this knowledge, or "strength of self," gives you a confidence that is very attractive. Remember, energy is magnetic, if you can fall in love with yourself, so will everyone else.

So hold on to your power. Loving yourself takes energy, and vibrational remedies are there, ready and willing to help. In addition to the suggestions in this chapter, see the chapter on using color in your environment to support your intentions.

Color Prescriptions for Loving Yourself

Just as green represents the heart chakra on the physical level, pink is said to represent it on the spiritual level. Intuitives able to see chakra colors often see pink surrounding the green heart chakra. **So surround yourself with both GREEN and PINK to strengthen your self-love.**

Give yourself a green or pink Color Shower (page 78). Envision yourself immersed in pink, floating peacefully in the universe.

Take a pink color energy bath (use a red color bath available in health food stores to turn the water pink). While you are bathing, really experience yourself physically, allow your hands to caress your body. You'll be absorbing the healing pink energy, as well as honoring your body. Touch, including self-touch, is very important. It is healing.

Create your own "I love myself" ritual. Whether it's meditating on this thought and visualizing either green or a deep pink color or just looking in the mirror every morning and saying out loud to yourself "*You* are a superstar." You will be creating the vibration that increases your self-love as well as attracting love from others.

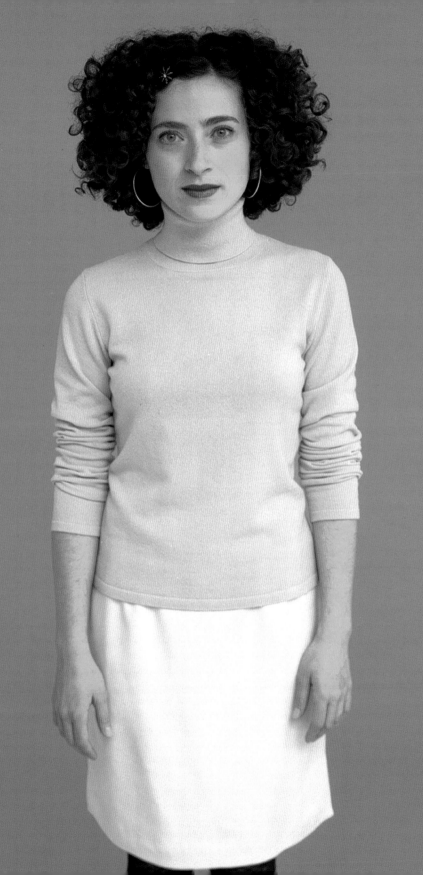

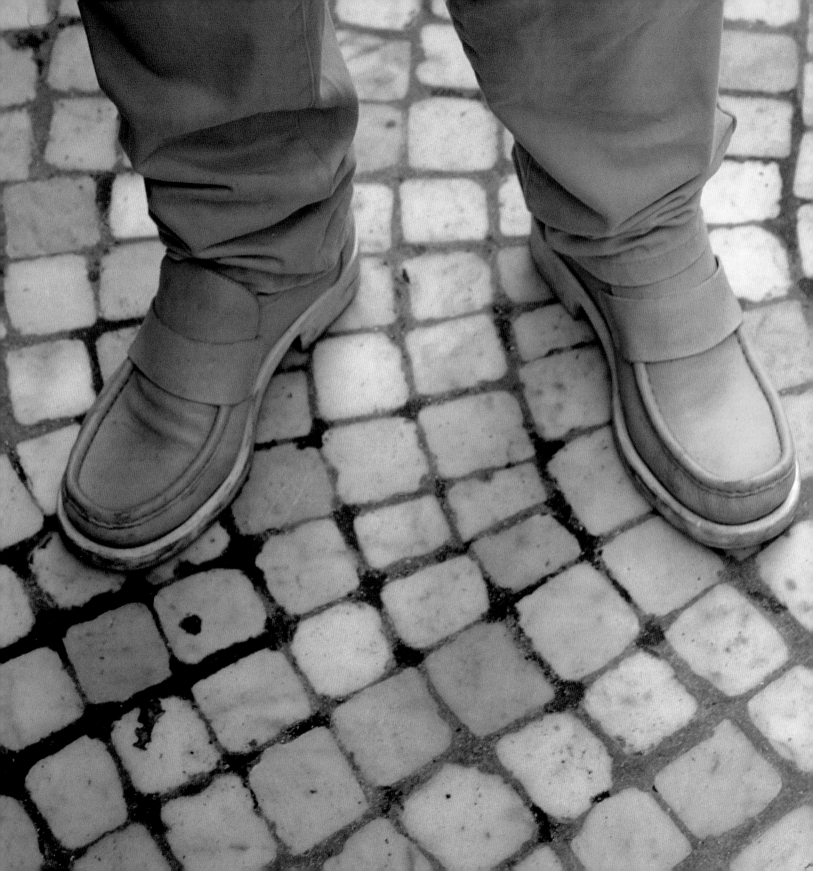

A few years ago I was feeling low and got to thinking that if time and space really is an illusion, as Dr. Robert Monroe suggests in his book *Far Journeys,* I could technically send myself healing energy from my future or past. So I just started sending myself love energy from my past. I loved my memories as if they were my children. Then, a day or two later, showering and still feeling a bit low, I felt this wave of warmth come over me. I almost felt giddy, and I thought, "Oh, this is my future self sending me positive energy." I usually see love energy as the color pink, but this energy seemed white. So now, whenever I need it, I ask my future self to send my present self a helping hand.

Finding Love

Feeding yourself the proper colors when you are single is crucial. Create an enchanted environment for yourself. I surround myself with lots of plants and flowers for fresh life force. I have lots of BLUES to ease loneliness, **lots of GREEN to promote self-love** and PINK to attract affection. It's important to really try to keep yourself centered, because if your energy system is out of whack, you won't be able to attract the person you want.

The goal is to achieve a state of self-sustaining happiness. When you can feel complete on your own, two really great things happen: You are able to see yourself properly and make changes accordingly, and you fall in love with yourself because you see your essence, which is pure love and creativity. Once your focus is on personal growth and creativity, you appreciate yourself more. And when your self-esteem is high, you will attract a mate who is also full of positive energy.

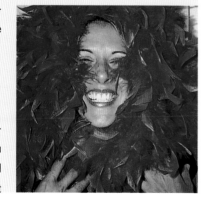

Color Prescriptions for Finding Love

Become a GREEN person. Surround yourself with green, wear it, visualize it.

Use PINK. Being a mixture of red and white, pink perfectly combines primal passion and purity. Hold a pink quartz and/or malachite crystal while you are meditating to clear your mind and heart. Keep the crystal with you at all times; it will put out the energy you want to attract. When the mind and heart

FINDING THE PERFECT MATE

Make a list of the qualities you would like your ideal partner to have, such as generous, good-humored, spiritual, etc. (We are not talking about physical attributes here.) Be honest. No one need see this list. It is just a way for you to clarify what you want.

Go down your list and tick off those qualities that you can honestly say you possess. The few that don't describe you are the traits you need to develop in yourself. When you make the effort to become what you seek, you will meet your match.

We gave this exercise to a woman who had picked green. She confessed to wanting a love relationship but felt hopelessly stuck in the memories of her past relationship. She told us how making the list made her realize what she was missing. When we saw her four months later, she told us she had immediately plunged into changing her life and was now engaged. She said she had let go of the past and never felt better about herself or more in love.

are cluttered, you are unable to register what your heart truly feels because you are caught up in whatever story the mind is repeating to you. The malachite crystal will help you to focus on the kind of person you want to meet.

Wear PINK—you'll absorb the color's therapeutic energy and also be making a statement that you are open to receiving and giving love. And wear pink makeup—it always gives a fresh, youthful look and the glow associated with new love.

Place PINK flowers in your bedroom and light a pink candle.

Use the White Bubble Technique (page 79) substituting PINK.

RED stimulates passion and will help you give off the right vibes. Wear red, especially undergarments. If you feel sexy you will be sexy. Red nails and lips, too, imply sexuality and mystery. Visualize red running through you and sending out sexual energy. Envision you and the mate you desire surrounded by red sexual energy.

ORANGE connects us to our intuition, especially valuable in matters of the heart. Use it to trust your instincts about a relationship. If you've found a new love you're uncertain about, meditate on PURPLE, wear purple, and bathe in purple so that your third-eye chakra can connect you to your higher self to find out whether your new love interest is right for you.

Sometimes we want to enter a new relationship but we're really not ready. As you work on yourself, remember that being without a partner does not have to be an unhappy time. A YELLOW candle will bring joy, whether you are with someone or not.

 Being single has some very special pitfalls, like meeting someone, deciding he (or she) is the one, and becoming infatuated. Whenever I feel I'm holding on too tightly to thoughts of me and a guy, I try to stop and take time out to balance myself. I light a sage stick (a bundle of dried sage sometimes mixed with lavender and other herbs available where herbs are sold). Once it's smoking, I walk around the apartment with it to cleanse the atmosphere, especially the bedroom. When the preoccupation I feel is intense, I buy white flowers and put them in my bedroom for more cleansing.

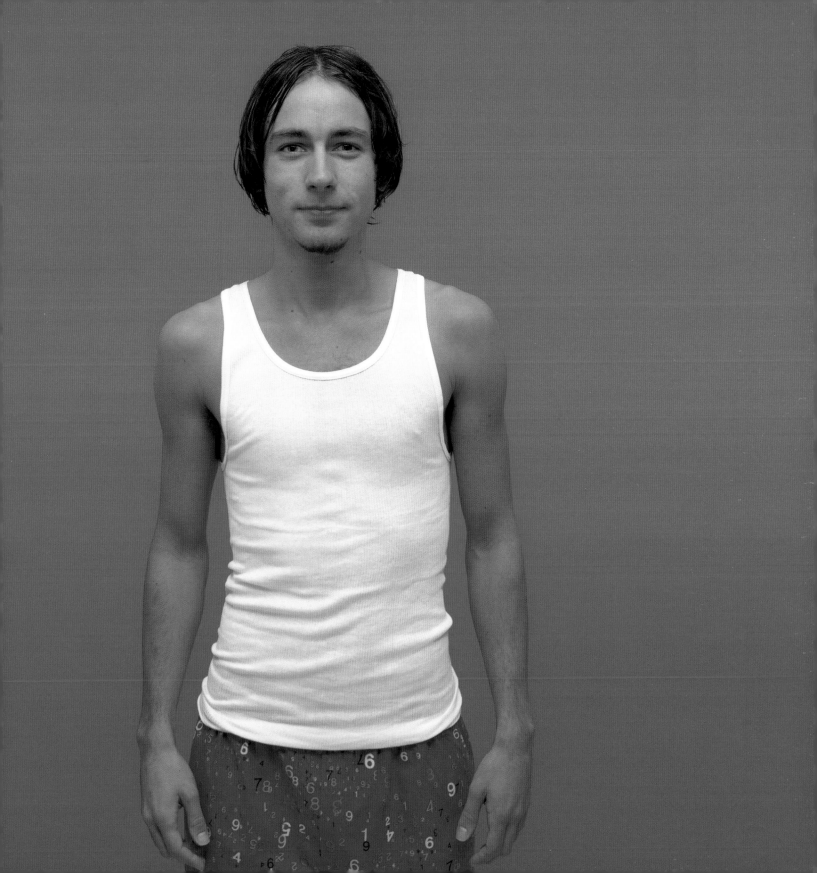

Next, I carve out a few hours so that I can spend time with myself. Solitude is different from being alone. I have fun. I write, I paint, and I usually always end up in some wonderful daydream (a visualization really) about being strong and happy and having the relationship I want. But I'm careful to be nonspecific. I acknowledge that the person I feel connected to is the person I might be wanting now, but this could change at any moment. Being open to when a relationship is right and when it's wrong is extremely important in a single girl's life because you may want a relationship but you may not be ready. Knowing that is important.

Loving a Partner

A relationship with a loving partner is the deepest, the most intimate love there is. It creates a true energetic exchange. The trust that allows two people to be open with each other, to share everything, and to be vulnerable forges a major bond. Many mystics and intuitives who have second sight can see an actual cord between two people who are in love. There's an energetic bond that connects them at the solar plexus, and the stronger the relationship, the stronger the cord. So when you hear a friend talking about how he or she feels so "connected" to a partner, what's being referred to is a real energetic connection. In healthy relationships the energy flows back and forth in a reciprocal fashion, but when the energy isn't returned, the person holding on becomes drained and the person who has disengaged feels invaded. When the relationship dissolves, it takes some time to disconnect—this is a major reason why we experience such grief when a relationship doesn't work out.

To strengthen the cord and keep your relationship strong, you want to make sure you are keeping your solar plexus, or YELLOW, chakra balanced. **Yellow helps your self-esteem and confidence, which in turn helps you maintain an equal relationship with a mutual exchange of energy.** You don't want one person draining the other. If either you or your partner feels insecure, you need to employ yellow energy techniques. You'll also want to feed yourself and your partner green color energy to make sure you hold no resentments toward each other.

Miscommunication is a killer in relationships. **You want to surround yourselves in BLUE once in a while to make sure you are having honest and effective communication.** You'll also want to

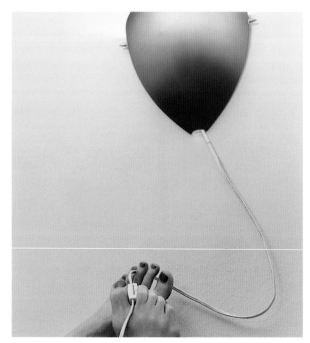

make sure you spend time in situations that allow you to drop your social masks, open yourselves to each other and nurture each other. GREEN, PINK, LIGHT BLUE, and WHITE are all colors that can support this process. If you live together, make sure your living space includes GREEN for love, ORANGE for sexuality, BLUE for honest communication, WHITE for cleansing, and something BLACK in the living area. Black will promote forward movement, help to discourage you from becoming *too* comfortable with your partner, and keep your relationship fresh.

Color Prescriptions for Loving a Partner

Wear RED lipstick and lingerie to stimulate mutual passion. Buy red flowers for the bedroom and/or the love area of your home. Buy red sheets. Use them only for passionate nights, not when you have to be up early. Use a red lightbulb for mood lighting and/or rose or jasmine-scented votive candles. Imagine red coursing through you while you make love.

When you want to have a serious discussion, light an ORANGE candle. Orange aids communication between two people who need to open up and work through an emotional process together.

Fill yourself with GREEN love energy in order to properly love yourself and your partner. Love must be nurtured. Take a green color bath, maybe together. Buy green sheets to promote unconditional love. Imagine green surrounding you while you make love. Paint the walls of the area where you and your mate do most of your talking together green for unconditional love; add traces of BLUE for communication.

When you need to make decisions involving your partner, use VIOLET. The violet color energy allows you to look at your partner and your situation objectively so that you can see clearly.

If arguments erupt, use WHITE to clear away any blocks and negativity that has built up between you. White will also protect you from any negativity coming from your partner. Check your bedroom to make sure it is clear of clutter and place some crystals in the room.

Color Prescriptions for Mending Love

When there is a rift in your relationship, the first color to think of is GREEN. Buy green sheets, wear green, visualize green, or paint with green. You will both need a lot of green to let go of past anger, resentment, and pain.

Use PINK to bring back the feeling of newness and create a healing atmosphere. When I find myself in a confrontational phone conversation, I hold a rose quartz in my hand. It really helps me to find love for the person I am arguing with, and that in turn usually helps end the fight.

Buy RED and WHITE carnations for the bedroom. Carnations absorb negativity.

Wear and visualize orange. **ORANGE allows you to see whether fixing the relationship is truly the best thing.** Sometimes relationships just aren't meant to be or they have beautifully served their purpose and it is time to move on. Your caring feelings don't have to change, just the form of the relationship.

Wear BLUE and sleep on blue sheets. Blue lets you speak your truth; without truth nothing can be truly mended. Truth can be painful, but if we learn from it and

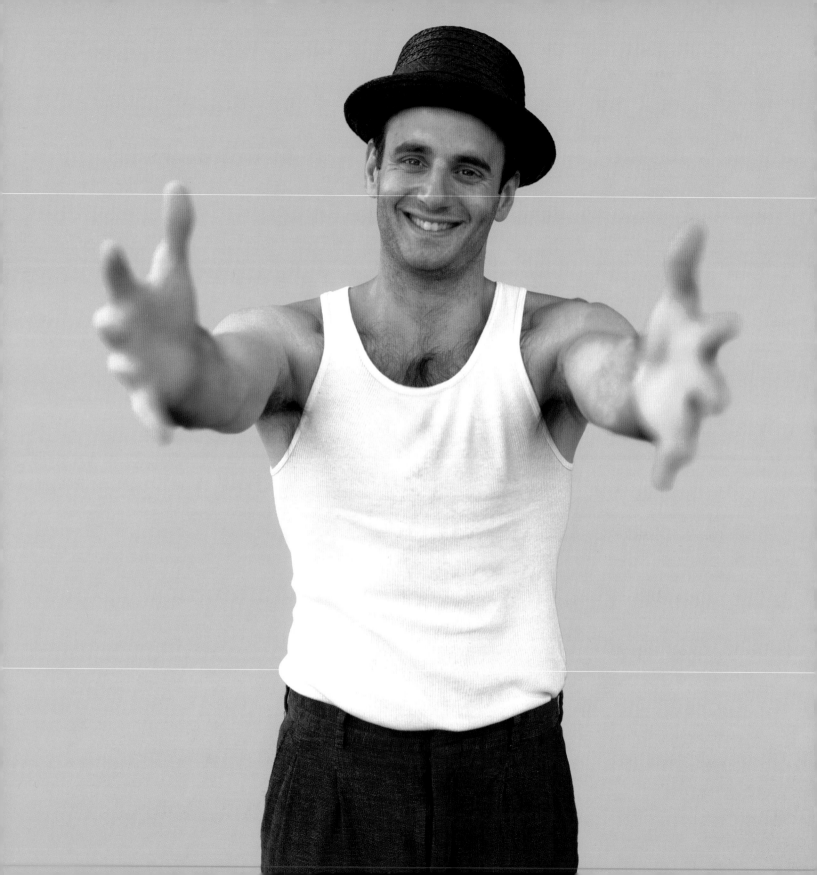

increase our self-awareness, we can break negative patterns. Visualize blue when meditating to help center yourself and focus on real issues.

Buy PURPLE pillowcases to help stimulate dream activity. When love is strained, dreams can help reveal the truth about the relationship.

Use WHITE to cleanse any past or present negativity. Wear it and visualize it. Use the White Bubble Technique (page 79).

Once the relationship is renewed, place something BLACK in your house that you will see every day to promote forward movement.

Color Prescriptions for Mending the Hurt When It's Over

The most important thing to remember is you're fine just as you are. Green will support you and help you to let go of any anger and resentment. Wear GREEN, visualize it, sleep on green sheets, put up green curtains, drink green Solarized Water (page 82). You can also use WHITE with the green.

When you meditate, visualize yourself as happy and full.

Hold a PINK crystal. Hold it as long as it feels good to you, as long as you feel drawn to it. Use the White Bubble Technique (page 79) substituting pink to connect your ideal happy and joyful self with the abundance of the universe so that it can physically manifest. See yourself as joyous without your past lover.

Visualize ORANGE to help you connect with your intuition to figure out what really happened and why, so you can accept that your breakup is for the best.

Blue will ease your loneliness and calm you down. Wear BLUE. Visualize it. Sleep on blue sheets. Put up transparent blue curtains that allow the light coming through to solarize your bedroom. (This can be done with any of the colors.) Assess the two of you truthfully; realize that maybe you weren't really your true self in the relationship. Let the blue energy help you reclaim your truth.

VIOLET will reconnect you to your higher wisdom, allowing you to see the big picture.

Use WHITE to cleanse yourself of the past. Wear it and buy white carnations for your bedroom. Use a sage stick to cleanse your environment of any past energy associated with the old relationship. It will create a good flow of new energy around you.

"One of the things I remember about my childhood is that the color of my room was apple green. That color has always been comforting to me and now (by choice) it is the color of my office, the color of my cell phone cover, the color of my luggage (well, the luggage is a darker green), the color of my toothbrush, and was the color of my car when I had one."
—Jamie

Love and Sex

Sexuality, like everything else, is very strongly connected to color. The red and orange end of the spectrum is most directly related to passion and physical pleasure, as the red and orange chakras are the energetic centers of our sensual world—red controlling our physical body and orange our relationships and sexual organs.

In the Tantric tradition, sexual energy has long been revered as a vehicle for reaching higher states of consciousness. The base of the spine is the resting place of a dormant energy called *kundalini*. This energy is depicted in ancient texts as a serpent curled around itself three times with its tail in its mouth. It is said that with practice, using breathing techniques and the right concentration of sexual energy, a loving couple can "wake the snake," allowing the energy to travel up the spine to the crown, igniting a feeling of infinite bliss. The practice holds the added draw that even if you never achieve this state of transcendence, you won't feel as if you are wasting your time practicing.

Though red is the primary color of primal passion and procreation, and orange the color for sexuality and desire, they aren't always the colors a person needs to get in the mood to make love. Individual needs determine which color can be used to stimulate and heighten sexual feeling and response. For women especially, a loving feeling usually sparks erotic impulses and green or pink is often the most effective color to enhance passion. Some people are most aroused by the feeling of spiritual communion, and purple or white is their best choice. If you want to introduce any of these colors for

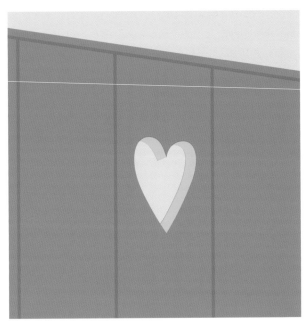

lovemaking, you can meditate on the color before making love, wear the color in question, or make sure the appropriate colors are part of the bedroom's decor. You can also visualize the color as you make love.

Many people report seeing various colors at the moment of orgasm. These colors generally reveal something about the person and his or her relationship. One woman we spoke to reported seeing blue. After some questioning, it became clear that it was only during lovemaking that she felt as though she was truly expressing herself and that her needs were being met. Another woman, in a long, especially loving relationship, reported regularly seeing green. **GREEN is about unconditional love for oneself and others.** When her auric field merged with her husband's, green was the color that reflected their love. A radiant pulsating white is another color that is commonly reported. White is associated with the divine, and because many people experience the sex act as a spiritual joining together, it follows that white would be the color they would see at the moment of climax.

One women we know who as a child had experienced inappropriate and misdirected sexual energy from her family also saw white when she came to orgasm. Since white is cleansing, she may have been instinctively feeding herself this color to cleanse her past emotional blocks. Also, the sex act itself can be very healing. Fun therapy.

Loving Friends

Love within friendship is highly underrated and underappreciated. We tend to forget the friends and colleagues around us who care about us and support us. We also put our relationships with our friends in a different category from our lovers and immediate families. Because they are so close to us, we devalue their positive influence. Female friendship is particularly filled with healing love energy. Women are usually good at friendship, and when they explore its emotional power, they find great personal satisfaction and strength.

When families and communities of friends intentionally create a positive loving environment for each other, their energy radiates to the broader community, and that in turn helps to positively influence the world. We all have the ability to have influential and meaningful exchanges, even if they are momentary. That's why all our daily exchanges are so important to the cosmic soup in which we swim daily, especially in cities. We must be very conscious of the energy we put out. All our actions should be in love.

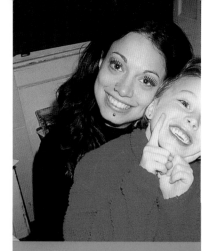

THE GIFT OF COLOR ENERGY
When shopping for a gift, consider what colors the recipient might need.
A sick friend: something red, yellow, or white to stimulate the immune system and lift spirits
A brokenhearted friend: something pink to fill the sense of emptiness with a sense of self, or green for self-love
An engagement gift: red or orange for passion; purple or white for a strong emotional bond
A wedding gift: silver for groundedness; green for unconditional love, white for looking forward, blue for honesty, red for passion
A new baby: green for unconditional love
A death: violet or purple to connect to the spirit of the person who has passed on

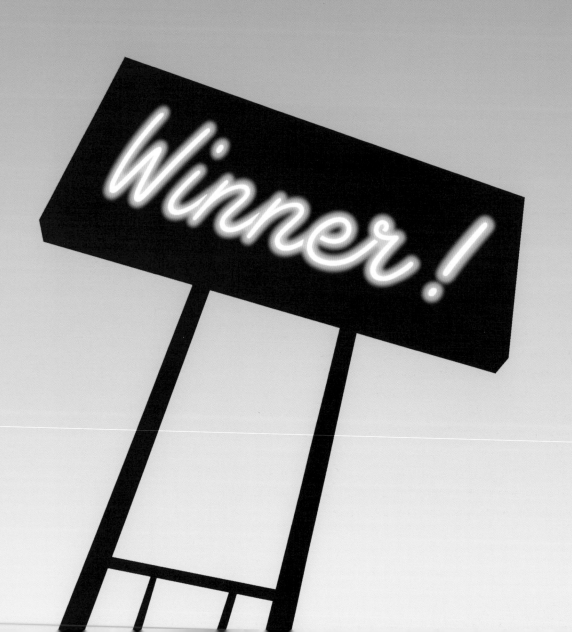

The Colors of Success

In the winter of 1996, Cristina and I were living together on the Lower East Side of Manhattan in a tiny studio with our bathtub next to our bed and an old gas stove next to the bath, a fridge next to that, and then you're back to the bed. To ward off the blues this cramped co-habitation seemed to bring on, we lined the bedraggled walls with our paintings and romantically imagined ourselves living in Paris at the turn of the century. We had been working toward our individual shows but looking at the vast amount of work all together, it seemed to have a narrative. It was like a garbled biography of our relationship. So we put all of our work up at the Gerswin Gallery in Chelsea and awaited our art stardom. The work ranged from my very pop-looking spirit guide paintings to the emotionally kinetic abstract paintings Cris had been making. When viewed together the general theme of the show was energetic, so we titled it Exorsted. One of the more throwaway ideas we developed was a color therapy nail polish set we called Cosmic Consciousness at Your Fingertips. It consisted of seven bottles of nail polish each filled with a different chakra color. Our concept was a critique on the cosmetic industry's lack of understanding of color and its true energetic nature.

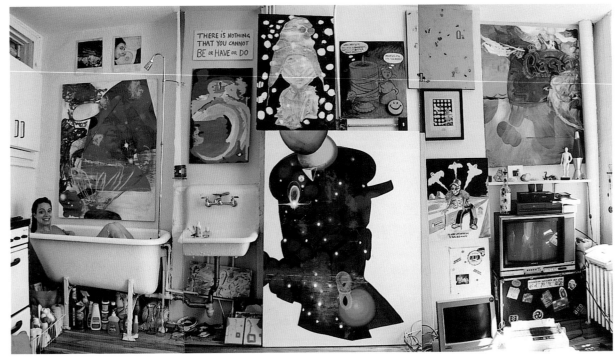

Well, *The New York Times* never made it to the show—in fact, hardly anyone but our core group did. So, with our tails between our legs, we retreated to Miami to Cristina's mom's for a cheap and desperately needed vacation. Cristina's mom had given us the book *Creative Visualization,* in which the author, Shakti Gawain, explains the magnetic nature of thought and how we create our reality according to the way we think.

Cristina and I discussed these ideas for hours and the excitement we felt gave us new hope. We decided that as an art experiment, we would completely accept the law of attraction and consciously apply it to our lives. Using a visualization technique from Shakti Gawain's book, we immediately set about shaping our future.

What did we want? We wanted to travel a lot together. We wanted artistic freedom. We wanted to make lots of money. We wanted the opportunity to speak to the world about color therapy and the implications of vibrational healing as a consciousness-raising tool. Then we imagined a big pink bubble; we placed our visualization of our perfect life in the bubble and sent it off into the universe. We did this with the strangest sense of certainty.

Three weeks later to the day we received a phone call from our friend Andrew, who had been talking about starting his own business. He wanted to know if we would be interested in creating a line of cosmetics as he had some contacts in the industry. At first we resisted, as cosmetics were something we saw as Old World and not part of our vision, until he reminded us of our color therapy nail piece. That's when the other shoe dropped. This was it! It was as if the concept was inventing us. Over the next months the three of us put together a business proposal, raised $250,000 from private investors, and started Tony&Tina Vibrational Remedies.

The universe has limitless abundance and offers success to us all. The universal pie is infinite. When we take a big piece, it doesn't mean that someone else will have to go without. So go for your heart's desire. Go for wanting it all. Our potential is limited only by our doubts. Putting doubt aside can be a challenge, but with practice, it becomes routine. We'll tell you how.

First, though, you need to get in touch with what it feels like to be open and aware of how things really make you feel. If you have an overriding feeling of happiness and energy, you're in a good place. But sometimes we stop noticing our feelings because we've gotten comfortable with the status quo. And sadly, some of us are so worn down by a situation or a person or an illness that we become paralyzed, justifying things, hiding from things. If you feel heavily stuck in the quagmire of life, you can revive your energy system and put it back in working order by looking to the chakras and the vibrational remedies.

Success requires that your energy flow through you freely so that you have a sense of groundedness, confidence, and ease. The throat and base chakras are especially important to success. Red, the base chakra, is associated with assertiveness, and blue, the throat chakra, is associated with effective communication, both of which are essential in any area of life but especially in the workforce. You need to be clear about what you want in order to get what you want. And to avoid miscommunication, you need to communicate in ways people understand.

Once you're on the path to understanding your energy system, you'll be on the road to health, happiness, and success. You'll start trusting your gut/intuition. You won't be afraid to change your mind or to make major life decisions because you'll know what your intuition is telling you to do. You'll be able to accept the messages you receive from your higher self and you'll find success in whatever way you are seeking it.

If You're on the Wrong Career Path

If you feel frustrated or unhappy or you lack energy and hate the idea of going to work at all, you are probably on the wrong career path or at least in the wrong work situation.

In this case, the first thing you need to do is cleanse yourself with WHITE. As we accumulate blockages or negativity, we are literally weighed down; we become heavy with our own self-imposed burden. You can wear white, which is easy to do. Sleeping in white sheets is effective because, during sleep our system is more receptive to absorbing energy. Most effective is a white color shower.

A friend of ours who had been with a company for

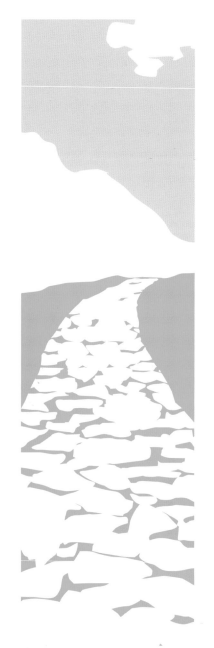

four years became more and more unhappy. Finally, things came to a head and he had to make a decision about whether to go or stay. He decided to go and made a clean break, opting to pursue his passion for art with all his energy. The week he cut the cord he connected with three different people who could help him in his new career. Energetically, he had made room and attracted what he really wanted.

When he told us this story, we reminded him that about a month earlier he had bought a white couch and that we had commented on his wearing more white—that white had helped him clear the obstacles from his path. He now had a newfound confidence about himself and seemed empowered. His gut had led him to the right path, reinforcing his own inner potential.

Wear ORANGE to strengthen your intuition and take an orange color shower. In order to get off the wrong path you need to realize you are on the wrong path. We often become habituated to our unsatisfactory situations and rationalize our duties. Orange energy will encourage you to listen to yourself and to reclaim your power. Our bodies always know the truth, we just have to listen. Orange energy will also fill you with the power to take action and move on.

YELLOW can also be helpful. Yellow increases self-esteem and inner power, which is what you need in order to recognize that you could be doing whatever you dream of doing. When we don't feel good about ourselves, we usually don't take active steps toward pursuing our happiness. Yellow will help you to take action.

Finding the Right Career Path

Use color energy to help support your system and fill you with positive energy. A clear energy field automatically raises the frequencies of your chakras and aura, attracting people who are in a position to help you and attracting a higher level of work. Be open to all possibilities. Even if a job situation seems inappropriate, notice how you feel when you think and talk about it. The right path may not be the one you had in mind. And remember, most of the time we don't think big enough.

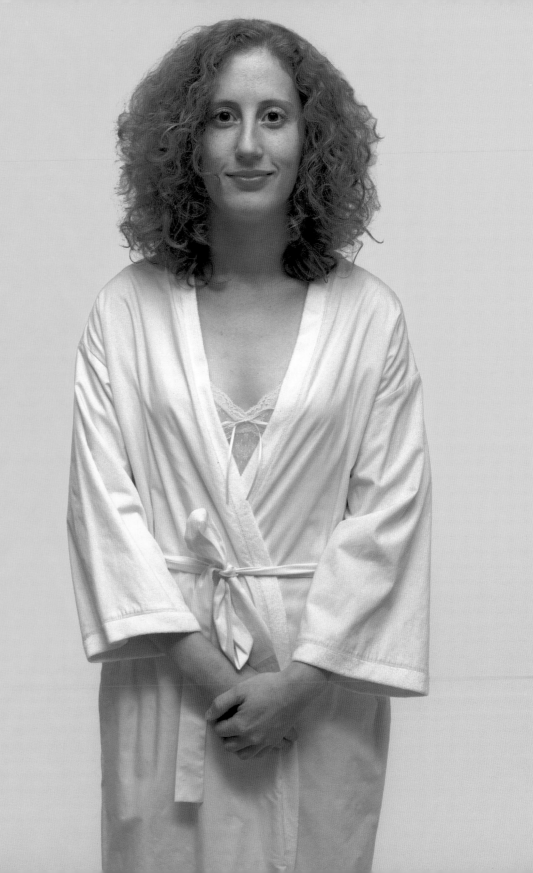

Wear ORANGE for intuition and give yourself an orange color shower.

Look at a YELLOW painting to stimulate your intellect.

Hold a GREEN malachite or calcite crystal to clear the clutter from your mind and to open yourself to messages from your heart about what path to take.

Do a color energy shower with PURPLE to connect with your higher self. Once you have access to your infinite wisdom you will always be guided the right way. The purple energy also allows us to see properly. If you're trying to find your way, detaching and seeing objectively is always a good thing. The purple energy promotes objectivity and protects you from seeing situations or people through a lens of fear or desire. You might be afraid of doing what you love because of money worries or preconceived notions of other problems, so let the purple wash away the perceptual clutter making way for clarity.

Finding Work

When you are looking for a job or deciding on a course of action, again, notice how you feel. The perfect job may be hidden in the guise of an imperfect one, preparing you for something not yet imagined. Or perhaps you know exactly what you want to do but you let doubt get the better of you. By allowing yourself to feel doubt, you are essentially putting out energy to ensure that you don't get what you want. Color can help clarify your ideal job and support the manifestation of it.

Use the PINK bubble technique to launch your desires into the universe. Suspend your disbelief, pretend you're at the movies. Believe for that moment it's all real, it's all present. We recently felt we needed some extra *oomph*. Tony had a red balloon left over from his birthday so we held it out the window, visualized new ideas coming to us, and launched it off into the universe. The moment we did this, we felt a difference in the energy surrounding us. The manifestation had begun. A concrete visual really helps to make it real.

Meditate, visualizing yourself in your ideal job incorporating GOLD and PURPLE, as they both help manifest thought into physical form. See the purple and gold surrounding you in your perfect job, empowering you to shine.

Cleanse yourself using WHITE to prevent any subconscious negativity from getting in your way.

Getting Through the Interview

Wear RED undergarments to bring out your assertiveness and courage. But don't wear a red or bright pink power suit—it's too aggressive and may turn off whomever you are trying to impress.

Wear BLUE, maybe a scarf or tie, which places the color right on the throat chakra so its benefits are felt immediately. Not only will it aid effective communication, crucial to success, but it will help instill personal integrity.

Wear ORANGE somewhere on your person for heightened intuition and burn an orange candle in your career area the night before to aid in your positive communication.

Give yourself an orange and YELLOW energy shower before the interview to increase your intuitive skill and stimulate your intellect in sussing out the situation and knowing how to act. Our insecurity and eagerness to impress can often cause us to come across as stiff and awkward. The intuition power of orange and the intellectual power of yellow will help guide you in the nonverbal aspects of the interview.

Starting a New Job

Cleanse yourself with WHITE so that you are entering your new post without any baggage. Use GREEN for this purpose as well. Green will allow you to let go of any resentment or anger—two things you definitely don't want to take with you. Let this new move be a fresh start. Present your ideal self and you will become your ideal self.

Wear BLUE to communicate effectively. Miscommunication is a killer. It can really lead you, a coworker, staff member, or boss into negative feelings for no reason. So be clear and honest with the people around you.

Wear green to stimulate your heart chakra and help you to be open and loving to the new people and situations you will be encountering.

Burn a YELLOW candle and meditate, visualizing yourself happy in your new job/career. Wear something yellow so that your mind will be sharp. You can even wear a red string around your finger to remind yourself that you are safe, strong, and powerful.

Burn an ORANGE candle during the first week and wear something orange to help your intuition guide you toward joy and wisdom.

Accepting Abundance

Abundance manifests through money, love, self-fulfillment, and happiness. What makes us happy will, in turn, make us abundant. Expect and be grateful for the abundance you will receive.

Be wary of what we call poverty consciousness—the belief that if you have more, someone else has to have less. This is not true. It is the nature of the universe to be abundant. Poverty consciousness is extremely negative and attracts exactly what you don't want. When you visualize yourself as needy and without, the universe will promptly respond and give that back to you.

Wear WHITE to cleanse yourself of negativity. We talk a lot about cleansing yourself of negativity and that's because this one idea is at the heart of everything. Negativity takes up space inside you, creating obstacles to what you want. If you don't let go of it, you can't see that you can have what you want, that you can attract the people and situations you want to attract. So white is a very important energy to connect with on a daily basis, and especially during times of change and turmoil.

Use ORANGE and PURPLE to find your intuition and higher spirit. When trying to connect with the universe, a colleague of ours imagines a bluish/purplish tube connecting him to his limitlessness. He then feels confident that anything he wants can be his.

Use RED and BLUE to put your thoughts into action and communicate effectively. Buy fresh white and red carnations to absorb negativity.

The Success Map

Mapmaking has brought great things to everyone we know who does it. We learned about this visualization technique from Shakti Gawain, who encourages mapmaking as a way to consciously bring about events. To test the idea out, we had everyone in our company make a huge map with their photo in the middle surrounded by images and affirmations representing their desires for their personal future. We all had our maps by our desks in the office, charting our respective courses. As most people wanted to be more successful in their jobs, doing this also served the company, breathing life into the organization and empowering everybody.

How to Make a Map

Take a large piece of paper, at least eleven by fourteen inches, or buy a piece of white cardboard. Gather up your materials—photographs, magazines, scissors, felt-tip markers, a glue stick or rubber cement, paint, whatever. Look through the magazines and cut out the images of those things you want to bring into your life. Cut out key words from headlines, too. Paste everything down. Draw or paint. Don't hold back. Make this a pictorial collage of your wishes come true.

One woman we know made a success map years ago and recently discovered it in a bureau drawer. Every one of her images had become reality.

When I look at all the maps I've made, I'm always amazed that they document major events in my life before they happen.

I keep my success map on the wall of my bedroom and look at it every morning and evening.

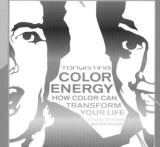

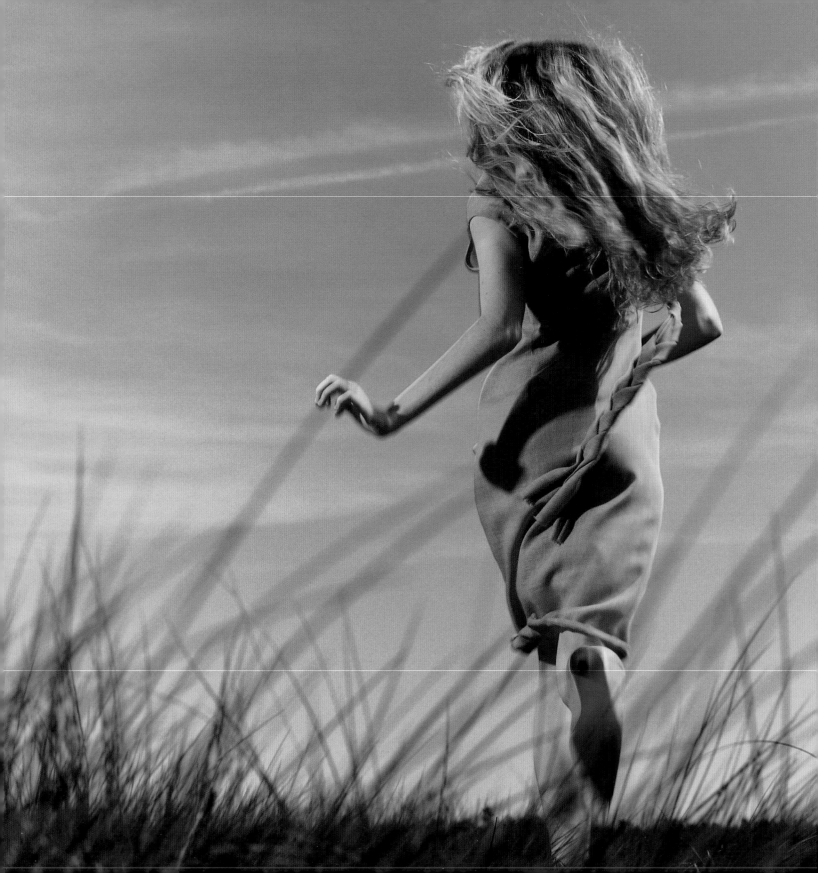

Color Medicine

Sometimes, when we feel at one with our true sense of self and with everything and everyone, we fill up with a definite knowing, a happiness that makes us feel like there's a summer breeze that's just passed by and a lightness that lifts us off the ground. That feeling, somewhere between happiness and tears, lets you know you are really connected. For most of us, this feeling is fleeting. It comes and goes. So when you get a hint of something fitting this description, just register it and remember it as a sensory memory. When you suspect you are connecting, you are ready to heal your body, mind, and spirit.

In a sense, we have been talking all along about color medicine and vibrational healing with color. In this chapter we focus more specifically on healing particular conditions.

There are many ways to heal, but the most important element necessary for true healing to occur is being open to the idea that you can heal. We must want to heal and believe that we deserve to heal. We're all so impatient; we're all so skeptical, we visualize our dis-eases as beyond our control. (Doubting is visualizing; sorry, that's the hard part.) We are the only ones who can truly heal ourselves. A doctor can surgically remove a tumor, but he can't remove the negative vibration that created the environment that enabled the tumor to grow. Only you can do that by having a balanced, healthy, and cleared energy system.

If you are out of balance, you unwittingly send out negative intention that eventually circles its way back into your life as some unwanted symptom or emotion. Our experience is that negative intention usually presents itself as a fear. Then, because you are afraid and worried, you begin to obsess, which fuels the fear. The fear then manifests in a physical way. You see the cycle. To become healthy and to stay healthy we need to balance our energies to effectively create positive manifestations.

 Ever since I was a child, I had a feeling that there was more to illness and disease than met the eye. From as early as I can remember, I suffered from hypochondria, fueled by my mother's continual lament that I was "coming down with something." When she said these words, even though I felt fine minutes before, I would slip into the flu or something equally debilitating. It is now clear to me that those years were my training ground for being a generally sickly kid.

I grew up in a council estate in south London in a family more often on welfare than wages. All the kids I knew were from low-income homes, but one family in particular stood out as being really poor. We all referred to the children from this family as Gyppos, a derogatory term for Gypsies. (Actually, this term would have been better applied to me, as my grandfather was the first in our family to live in a house rather than a caravan.) These Gyppos were a constant source of amazement to my parents as, even in winter, they would go around in T-shirts and bare feet. My mum would comment daily that one of these days "they'll catch their death." As I watched them playing out in the rain from my sickbed, it became clear to my ten-year-old mind that this was not the case. Actually, they were pictures of radiant health. One time after school I ran into the oldest of the boys as he was trying to steal some handlebars from a bike. The temperature was in the fifties and he was topless.

"Ain't you cold?" I ask.

"No. Well, yeah," he grunts, absorbed in his task.

"Won't you get sick?" I wait impatiently as he untwists the last few threads of a bolt.

"Cold don't make you sick, it makes you tuff," he says.

"How come?" I persist, and his answer is the first epiphany in my ten confused years.

"My dad told me."

This kid's parental conditioning had been as strong as mine with exactly the opposite message. Even though I had never heard the word *affirmation,* from that day on I began to reprogram myself with authoritative statements. My favorite one then was "There's just something about you that makes girls want to talk to you." And when Mum started in on her sick stuff, I would play my own message in my head: "I feel really good."

Holism

The holistic health movement has embraced the concept that no aspect of self can be successfully treated unless it is considered as part of the whole, that all four elements of our energetic system—physical, emotional, intellectual, and spiritual—are interdependent.

All sickness develops when our general energy system becomes weakened, and this is often related to emotional strife. When you do become ill, consider whether there is an underlying emotion, attitude, or spiritual belief that may have caused your illness or contributed to it. In this way your physical symptoms can guide you to focus on other aspects of your being in a very specific way. Look beyond your symptoms. For instance, you may become fatigued when you feel you are not getting the emotional attention or appreciation you need. Understanding this can lead you to deal with green issues of the heart chakra and unconditional love. Or, if you suffer from chronic bronchitis, you may see that you have a problem communicating what you really feel. Or your problem could be that you're vulnerable to addiction or do not have the willpower to make the choices you need to make. These are all issues of the blue throat chakra, which, when blocked and not properly dealt with, will inevitably manifest physically. Practicing and preaching are two different things. I, Tina, had a throat chakra issue that I ignored, and I developed tonsilitis three times in six weeks. I finally got it—I recognized it was time to consciously process my issues. I bought an aquamarine choker, wore it for two weeks, and felt my chakra strengthen and balance.

If you accept that good health is more than not being laid up in bed, you can logically understand why holism is essential. Many doctors today realize that there are emotional and spiritual components to disease and will attempt to address them or try to advise on complementary therapies. The biggest breakthrough has been in appreciating the effects of stress and recognizing when people need a break from it all. Our society has made "personal downtime" dirty words. We are always supposed to be doing something. Nothing is a good thing sometimes, as your doctor may tell you. The more we, as health consumers, demand holistic treatment, the faster change can take place.

The Three Essentials of Health

Controlled breathing, meditation, and yoga, disciplines developed thousands of years ago by monks to strengthen mind and body and lay the foundation for spiritual practice, are gifts we can use today not only to stay fit but to help pre-

"The Buddhist understanding is that it is primarily incomplete breathing that causes disease. If you breathe fully, you will be free of disease and you will begin to live harmoniously in the world. So I ask all of you to allow your breath to be full and deep and to relax yourself in your life."
— *Joshu Sasaki Roshi*

DEEP RHYTHMIC BREATHING
You can do your breathing sitting or standing. In either case, be sure that your spine is straight and your head erect.
1. Breathe in and really imagine that your breath is filling your body. Breathe and feel the air going in through the top part of your nose, traveling down your spine, and up again to fill your chest. Put your right hand above your navel and your left hand on your chest to become accustomed to this movement. Notice how full you can become. Gently release the breath from the chest downward. Your chest and stomach area will deflate. Really exhale all the way, allowing the toxins and carbon dioxide to flow out. This exhaled breath is heavier than an inhalation, and you will feel it exiting through the bottom part of your nose. Concentrate on relaxing your tongue with your jaw open and lips together.
2. Before you begin the next inhalation, just as a metronome pauses before it reverses direction, slow your rhythm for ↓

pare our bodies to receive color energy. If you make these practices a part of your daily routine, you will be amazed at the difference it will make to your life.

Breathing

The reason breath is so important is that it is our connection to the present. We all live mostly in a combination of the past and the future, both of which are easy for us to conceptualize. But the present cannot be conceptualized, it can only be experienced one breath at a time. As soon as we start to think about the present we are no longer in it. This is the trap. It is within this moment that all healing takes place. So concentrate on the breath and be here now.

When you breathe in positive energy and breathe out negativity and tension, you are creating an atmosphere in your energy system that is receptive to the vibrational effects of color therapy, aromatherapy, and positive thought. You will be putting yourself in a healing state. You can recover from depression, anxiety, and pain more readily because your energy will be flowing freely; you will not be energetically holding on to "this shouldn't have happened" and "that person is upsetting me." You'll breathe through this sort of mind chatter and move on. You'll enter a state of being with a higher frequency that allows you to rise above guilt and blame and courageously accept that the world is our mirror and that we can create whatever we desire. Your breath will prepare you to receive the color and thought that will allow you to heal and change your life.

Meditation

Deep breathing leads naturally into meditation, where you allow your breath to settle into a relaxed rhythm of inhalation and exhalation. When you begin meditating, start with as little as five minutes a day and slowly build to fifteen. Eventually you'll want to do half an hour a day. Strive for a state that gently releases thought as simply as it comes. Be soft. Live an eternity in the increasing gap between thoughts. It is in this open space that you will know your true nature and learn that your true nature is divine.

In a deep state of meditation, you can experience space and time as

Using Color to Heal Physical Ailments

This chart will tell you which colors are useful in healing various physical, emotional, mental, and spiritual conditions. With a basic knowledge of color therapy and a trust in your internal wisdom and intuition, you can use color vibration to heal, align, and balance your energy system.

RED	Strengthens physical ENERGY. Helps ANEMIA. Helps alleviate COLDS, FLU, and BRONCHITIS. Influences REPRODUCTIVE SYSTEM. Aids CIRCULATORY SYSTEM. Helps CONSTIPATION and LISTLESSNESS.
ORANGE	Relieves MUSCLE STRAIN. Assists in FOOD ASSIMILATION. Helps GALLSTONES. Aids ELIMINATION. Boosts IMMUNE SYSTEM. Influences REPRODUCTIVE system. Helps MENSTRUATION problems. Serves to DETOX body. Helps ASTHMA, BRONCHITIS, COLDS, LUNG CONDITIONS, ALLERGIES, EPILEPSY, and GROWTHS.
YELLOW	Aids in the breakdown of FATTY ACIDS and STARCHES. Assists in MINERAL ASSIMILATION. Good for DIGESTIVE PROBLEMS and CONSTIPATION. Good for STOMACH. Promotes ULCER HEALING. Helps BLADDER, KIDNEYS, LIVER, and SPLEEN. Helps RHEUMATISM, DIABETES, and PILES. Relieves ALCOHOL POISONING.
GREEN	Influences THYMUS GLAND and IMMUNE SYSTEM. Activates GENERAL HEALING. CALMING to body. Helps ANXIETY and EXHAUSTION. Influences HEART, PULMONARY and CIRCULATORY SYSTEMS. Aids ASSIMILATION OF NUTRIENTS. Helps REGENERATION of tissue. Helps ULCERS, ASTHMA, HAY FEVER, BACK DISORDERS, COLIC, LARYNGITIS, MALARIA, and PILES.
BLUE	Very healing for CHILDREN. Helps HEADACHES and INFLAMMATION. Aids function of THROAT, ESOPHAGUS, MOUTH, TEETH, and THYROID. Helps LARYNGITIS. Affects RESPIRATORY SYSTEM and VOCAL APPARATUS. Helps prevent BALDNESS and CATARACTS. Helps COLIC, DIARRHEA, EPILEPSY, SKIN RASHES, and JAUNDICE. Light blue: HELPS ACNE and ANXIETY. Ice blue or aqua: helps BURNS, FEVER, and NAUSEA. Dark blue: helps ALLERGIES.
VIOLET	Influences the PITUITARY and ENDOCRINE SYSTEMS, and the IMMUNE SYSTEM. Affects the THROAT, ESOPHAGUS, EARS, and EYES. Helps CATARACTS. Helps ASSIMILATE MINERALS. Helps ALCOHOL poisoning. Helps lung problems: ASTHMA, BRONCHITIS, PNEUMONIA, and CONVULSIONS. Helps DIABETES, ARTHRITIS, and NERVOUS AILMENTS. Enhances SENSE OF SMELL.
WHITE	Affects NERVOUS SYSTEM. Affects SKELETAL SYSTEM and aids in BUILDING BONE. Aids BRAIN SYNAPSE activity. Helps RASHES and WOUND HEALING. Relieves COUGHING.

several seconds. When you reach this point in your breathing, it is as though time does not exist and you are fully in the present. 3. Let the breath become continuous and natural. In yogic practice, this is called Hum Sa breathing. Visualize your breath. Let your thoughts pass by like clouds. Feel negativity and tension draining from you. 4. Focused, deep breathing helps transform the air we breathe into energy. The thoughts we have during the breathing affect the vibrancy of the energy. Trust that you are doing it correctly and you will be doing it correctly.

Practice this in a quiet moment to get the rhythm and then start applying it in your daily life whenever you feel stress or fear. At the Pura Vida Yoga Center in Costa Rica, the breathing is done standing and is called Standing Wave Breathing. I, Tina, find it the most effective breathing technique I've ever tried, and after practicing it, I see a fundamental change in my approach to things.

illusions. You can understand that everything is connected, that nothing is separate from you and nothing within you is separate from any other part of you. As you tap into universal consciousness, you can begin to accept your endless potential.

Yoga

Yoga, a system of exercises that massages the internal organs and affects the body on a cellular level, is the third essential.

Introducing these practices into your life is the single most important action you can take toward combating stress and having a true understanding of reality. They help you know yourself and understand why you do what you do. And they condition your body and mind to be receptive to subtle energies, especially color.

Healing Others—The Four Essentials

Before you begin healing another person, you need to prepare yourself with these essential steps. Always feel free to moderate any of our suggestions; trust your internal wisdom to guide you to do what you have to do in the way only you can do it.

Ground Yourself

Visualize a strong cord coming out of your tailbone and see it anchored to a large stone or crystal in the middle of the earth. This is a powerful visualization that will leave you feeling energetically grounded.

Protect Yourself

Contrary to popular belief, we do have a choice as to what kind of energy we surround ourselves with and allow into our system. To protect yourself from unwanted or negative energy, visualize a white light forming a protective suit/bubble around your body/being. Intention is everything, so repeat this affirmation: "I will not accept any negativity, I am protected by universal love and light."

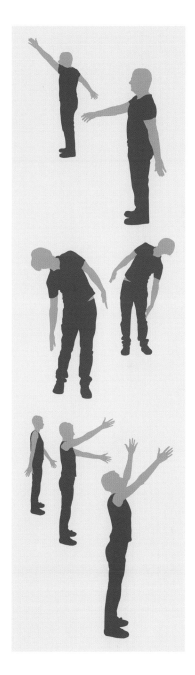

Cleanse Yourself

Cleansing is especially important when you are working on someone else. You don't want to bring any negative energy into the healing or take any with you when it's over. There are several ways to do this.

1. Visualize a rainbow showering down into the top of your head, washing through your body and passing out your feet.

2. Use a sage stick to cleanse yourself and your environment.

3. Soak in a bath with Epsom salts (use two cups to a tub of water).

4. Let your wrists go limp and shake your hands up and down for a few minutes.

5. Before and after a healing say to yourself, out loud if possible: "I am releasing all negative, unwanted, and blocked energy."

Balance Yourself

You can balance in many different ways.

1. Balance your male/female energies (page 75).

2. Picture each chakra, starting with the red base chakra, spinning three times to the left, then three times to the right.

3. Affirm to yourself that all your chakras are balanced and working harmoniously.

Cleansing Your Aura

1. Standing straight, hands by your sides, palms facing in, begin to slowly swing your arms in tandem forward and back. Let your arms slowly increase the arc of your swing. You should begin to feel as if your energy is being massaged around your thighs as your hands move past them. Once you feel this, begin to slowly decrease your swing until your arms have come to a stop.

2. Slowly bend to touch your knee on one side and then the other as if you have weights in your hands. Begin this shifting motion slowly, increase your speed, then decrease your speed and stop.

3. Place your palms facing each other in front of your lower belly and begin to make chopping motions, hands moving opposite each other. As you con-

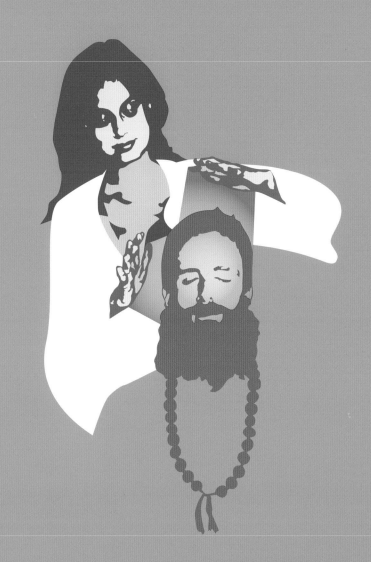

tinue this movement, begin to raise your hands up along your body following them with your eyes. When your hands are above your head, breathe in deeply and make a circular motion with your hands for three counts. Then reverse the direction of this motion while you breathe out.

Scanning

After preparing yourself for a healing, you need to assess what the other person (whom we will call "your friend") needs. Scanning is one method for discovering the blocks or weaknesses that need to be addressed. To scan, you allow your hand to roam lightly and freely over your friend's body along the chakras. By allowing your third eye to see into the body, you will sense the blockages.

 I did my first scanning spontaneously one night when Tony and I were hanging out. I suddenly got the urge to place my hands over his chakras. I shut my eyes and scanned his energy centers and discovered a block in his solar plexus chakra. I told him I thought he might need more yellow. The next week, our acupuncturist told him he was having spleen problems and needed to drink beet juice. The solar plexus chakra is associated with the spleen. I was amazed to learn I had been right. That I could scan was an amazing discovery for me and is something I continue to try to develop. We can all do this. We can scan and tune into how the energy feels. Just trust.

A Headache Healing

 A few years ago, when we began to realize that we were healers—as we all are—Tony and I created an intention—remember, intention is everything—to develop our healing abilities. About this time, Tony was having a really bad headache, which is unusual for him. So I said, "Well, blue is anti-inflammatory, so why don't I try projecting blue onto your head." As I said this, I immediately felt my hands heating up, an indication to me that my energy was being channeled directly into my hands.

I did the Four Essentials for Healing. Then I put one hand about six inches away from Tony's forehead and the other about six inches above his head, slightly toward the side. I shut my eyes and imagined a dome over my head, opening up to the universe. I then visualized blue light from the universe flowing down into my head, through my arm, and shooting out my hands into Tony's head. After a minute or two, he said, "Wow, this is really working!" I got a bit flustered. I was struggling with self-doubt and Tony immediately asked what had changed. I told him it was my doubt. So I refocused and in a few minutes his headache was gone. It was an amazing experience, and it reinforced for me how crucial belief and intention are to any healing.

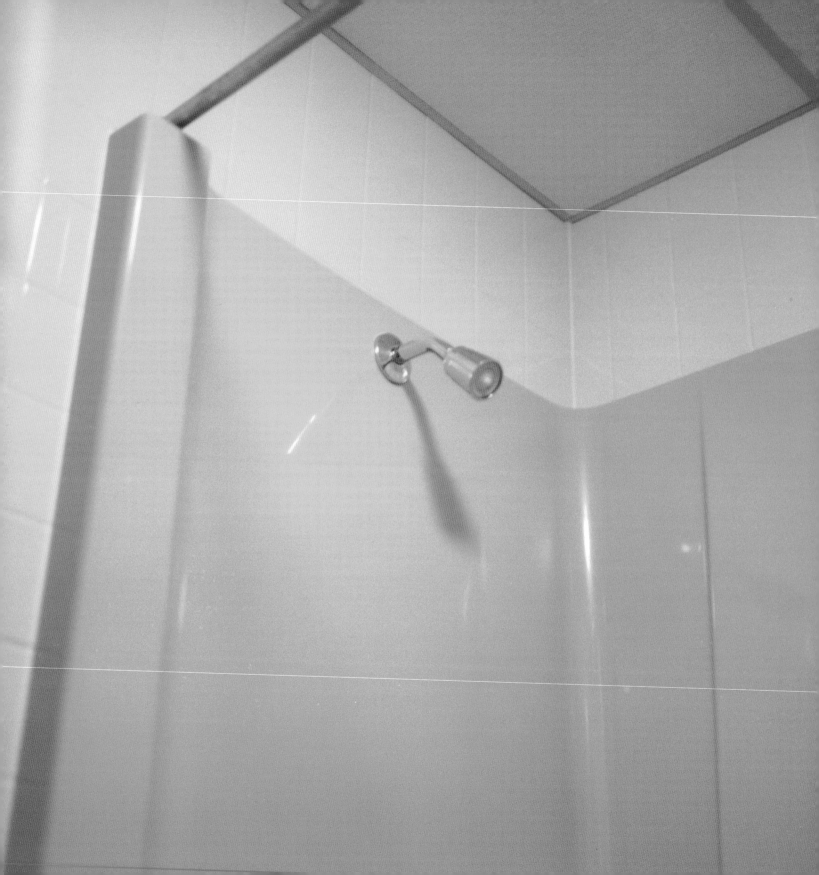

Rooms to Breathe In

Our home is our haven, our retreat. It's where we see our mate, family, and friends, and where we spend time alone. It's where we can let our hair down, relax, celebrate, entertain, meditate, plan, reminisce, eat, sleep, love. It is our spiritual center. It has nothing to do with fashion. As an extension of our personal energy, it should remind us of where we want life to take us. If you long for simplicity, then your home should reflect that. If you are on a spiritual path, then let your home set the stage. Begin by creating an enchanted environment for yourself. You want to feel calm and happy here and you'll find that by using color in a deliberate way you'll be making your home energetically supportive—a joyful backdrop to your life.

There are not many rooms that take more than three days to paint, and it is well worth it. Few symbolic fresh new starts are more powerful than changing the color of your room. We have personally found this to be the way out of many funks that can make the difference between feeling depressed and inspired. Changing the frequency of your environment changes the frequency of your situation. Also, the commitment to, for example, painting a bedroom in a

In ancient times there were many good-luck symbols to bless a household, and color was significant in each. In Ireland, Syria, India, Mexico, and Constantinople, the symbol of the red hand was used on a wall or door to shield the occupants from harm. In Jerusalem, a blue hand was used for the same reason.

shade of green to energize your heart center and work on matters of love is exactly the kind of affirmation it takes to set growth in motion.

There are a few other basic axioms to keep in mind to change the vibrational energy of your home.

• Get rid of clutter. It disturbs the mind on an unconscious level, lowering your tolerance for others and preventing you from radiating your inner light and joy.

• Avoid poverty consciousness. Hanging on to possessions because you feel you never have enough promotes stale stagnant energy. Release and let go to allow new energy to come into your life.

• Be thoughtful about the objects with which you surround yourself. This is not a question of economics, it is a question of choosing things that are meaningful to you. If you don't like an object in your house, it has to go, no matter how much it cost or who gave it to you.

• Take care of your home. When we take care of our surroundings we instantly enter a new state of awareness. Like Eastern monks tending their meditation gardens, we have a sense of satisfaction when we have undertaken and completed a project. The forward movement keeps us in the present, opening up our crown chakra.

• Cleanse. Use a sage stick to cleanse the house regularly and bring in fresh energy.

Making Color Choices

We'll tell you what we know, but you also need to check your intuition. Shut your eyes and ask yourself what color does this room need? As you develop your sensitivity to subtle energies and begin to trust your instincts, you will find that they will never steer you wrong.

Red

Use red judiciously as an interior color because it evokes a very powerful response. It also makes a room appear smaller. When you want coziness and intensity, as perhaps in an entry hall or dining room, red can work well. And while it may be great to make love in a red bedroom, sleeping would be out of the question. Red in the bathroom is great for your morning shower to give you courage in starting your day, but perhaps not so welcome when you want to relax in the tub. Burgundy, however, is fine.

Because red activates our base emotions and primal instincts, it can cause us to act thoughtlessly or aggressively. We saw (and heard) the results in the bar downstairs from our apartment. Fights broke out so frequently the place was about to be shut down. When we went in one day to comment on the latest uproar, we noticed that the pool table, the focal point of the space, was covered in red baize. We advised the owner to change it to green. To humor us, and perhaps out of desperation, he did, and to his amazement the fights almost completely stopped. So if you are living with red and find yourself prone to arguments and spats, change this color or balance it with golden yellows or greens.

One red story I found especially touching was about a woman suffering from postpartum depression. Not feeling sexy was her biggest complaint. She told me that about three months after her daughter was born she had the urge to paint her bathroom red. I wondered if she was subconsciously setting up a love nest for herself and her husband. The answer, to my surprise, was no. This was her place. She would spend hours in there rebuilding her sense of self and her sensuality. As her depression began to lift, she painted the window frames orange and yellow. She was rebuilding herself from the base chakra up.

Orange

Orange, which also connotes strong feelings, has some of the same limitations as red for interiors. Because it stimulates appetite, orange is commonly used in fast-food restaurants, as is yellow. For the home, it needs to be used sparingly. For example, in our first apartment, we had an old, unfashionable couch that looked terrible. We bought an orange sheet to cover it hoping to lift our spirits. It seemed all right at first until one day I, Tina, was overcome with the urge to get rid of it immediately; I was having a fit. Tony admitted that he'd been feeling antsy, too, so in no time, the orange sheet became curtains. The smaller amount of orange worked well on the windows, creating a subtle glow in the morning light that encouraged activity. As for the couch, we covered it with a pale blue throw and were much happier—and calmer. All mistakes are just experiences that help to teach us what is good or bad for us personally.

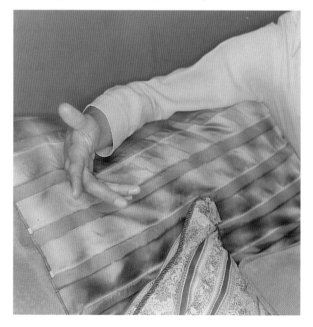

IF YOU DON'T WANT TO PAINT
If you want to change the color
energy in a room but find the
idea of painting your walls too
daunting, there are other possi-
bilities:
Just paint the door or window
    frames
Solarize the room with
    transparent silk curtains
Wear the color you need
Do color visualization
Do color meditation
Take a color energy shower
Place flowers in the room
Use colored sheets
Sleep with colored crystals

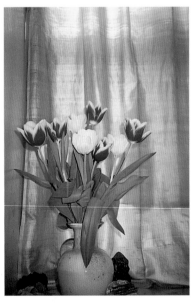

Yellow

Yellow is good for a room where you read and/or work. It's bright and uplifting, plus it stimulates the intellect and aids in strengthening your inner power
and self-esteem.

Green and Blue

Green and blue are great for promoting relaxation and sound sleep, so naturally they are the colors we recommend for bedrooms. One friend of ours was
suffering from insomnia. For months, she experienced a powerful urge to paint
her bedroom deep green, an impulse that surprised her because dark green
had never been one of her favorite colors. Eventually, she tried it and hasn't
had a night of insomnia since. Restful green was just what the doctor ordered.

Another friend, having recently suffered the loss of her father, felt com-
pelled to paint her bedroom blue. What she didn't realize at the time is that
blue eases loneliness. She was listening to her body's needs and benefiting
from soothing blue energy to relieve her grief.

Violet

Violet is a receding color and makes a room appear larger. Violet makes for a
contemplative living space, ideal for bathrooms and dreamy bedrooms. We
painted our bedroom area violet not only because it was very small but also
because violet helps stimulate dreams and spirituality. I (Tina) experienced an
increase in lucid dreams and from these dreams got inspiration for some of our
more unique nail colors. We would suggest painting a room violet when you
are going through dramatic emotional periods in your life. It will help your connection with the universe and inspire you to listen to your body and what it
needs.

White

Since white carries an otherworldly quality, it needs to be balanced with pictures, plants, crystals, and mirrors. White is a good choice when you want to
make a room appear lighter and/or bigger, as are all pastel colors.

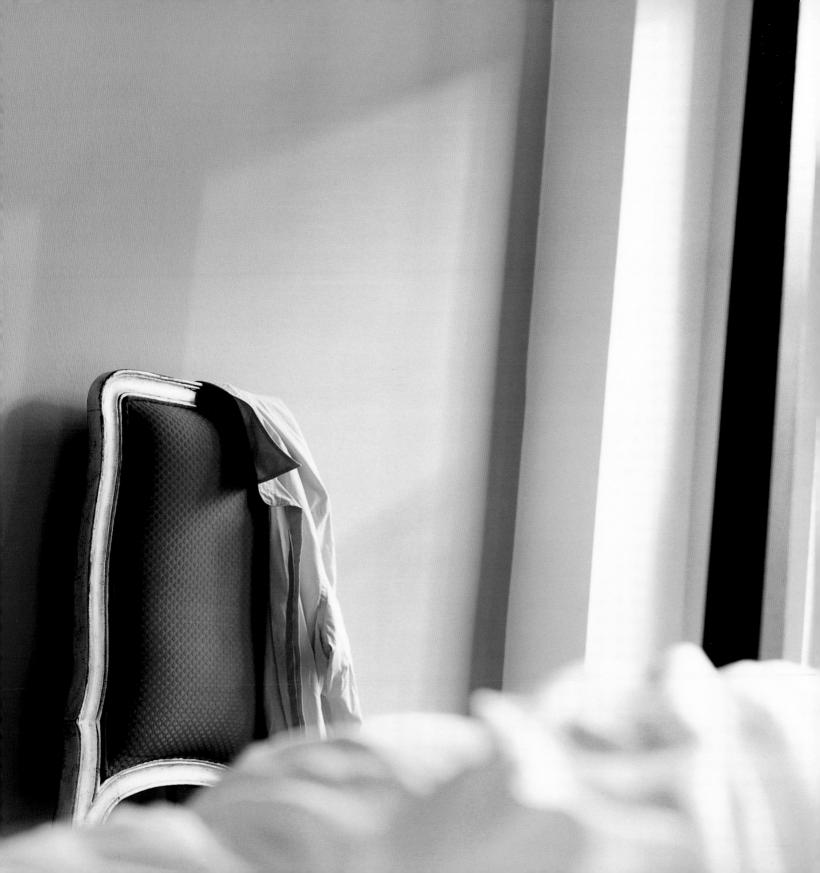

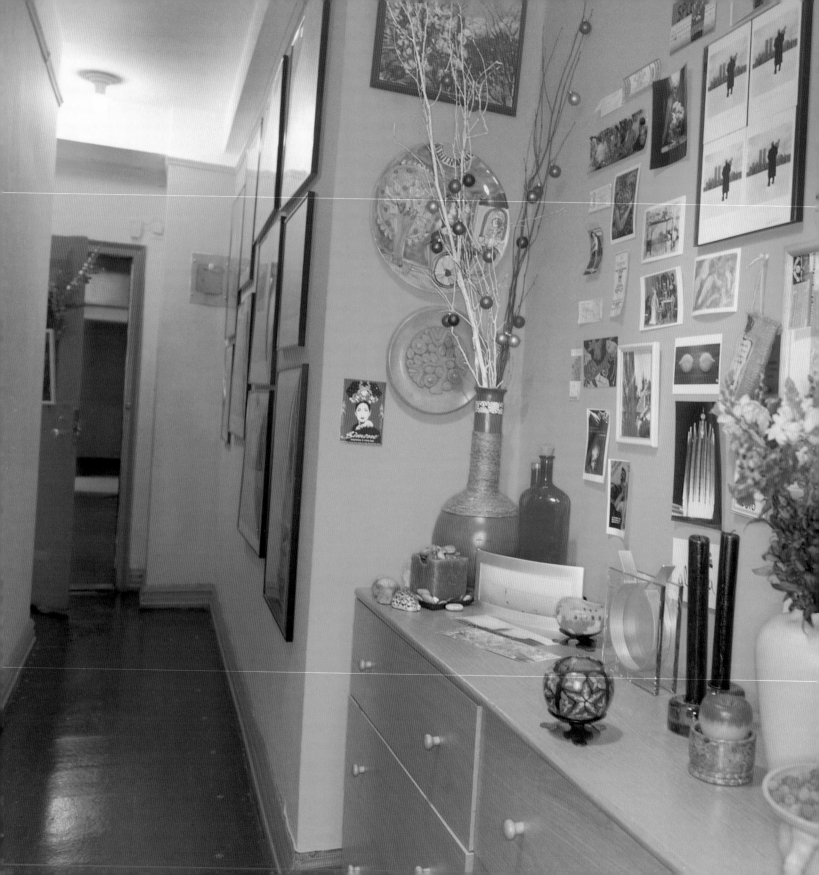

The Color-Correct Home

This blueprint for a vibrationally correct home will provide you with a starting point from which you may apply color in your own way. Use your intuition as well as our color guidelines for specific rooms.

The Entrance

First impressions are important. Red can indicate excitement and promise liveliness within. Blue may reflect a family with strong independent opinions. Green and pink announce warmth, perhaps a home where harmony and loving feelings are paramount. Yellow indicates a family where ideas and the intellect are valued. Hanging photographs of family and friends in the entrance can also remind you of the love in your life when you come home after a long day.

The Living Room

When you think about it, the words *living room* make a big statement since where and how we live affect our energy system and our overall happiness. Unfortunately, too many living rooms aren't lived in at all. We feel the living room should always have a welcoming, lived-in air and evoke a feeling of happiness and joy.

Warm colors are good choices for this room. Deep colors might make the room look smaller but they can have therapeutic effects as well. A deep burgundy might give a safe feel, a sexy feel. A burnt orange will promote sociability and sensuality and help bring conversations to an intuitive level. But in general, you'll want to go with calming colors for your dominant color. A blue will stimulate conversation and calm the nerves. Green and blue is a good combination because it promotes loving communication and relaxation. You can bring in bright and stimulating colors with paintings, flowers, pillows, loose throws, and vases.

Keep a strong and loving life force flowing in your home and especially in the living room. Plants are great for energy and aesthetics. Crystals can purify and stimulate conversation. Your own artwork on the walls can be a source of inspiration and conversation. Photographs of you in a special moment will remind you that you are loved and have achieved. Your living room should reflect your life.

The Dining Room

Since eating is a time for connecting with friends and family, effective honest conversation can be stimulated with blues, violet, or a muted orange mixed with a blue or green. Reds and oranges will encourage a more romantic, fiery mood. Eating can be a sensual time, so deep burgundies, deep violets, and greens or a burnt orange would work as well. It's interesting that the bright oranges used in fast-food chains promote sociability but don't say relax and stay a while, whereas a darker, more muted orange does. The same is true for yellow. Whatever color you choose, colored votives can really lend the room a magical light.

The Kitchen

For many people, the kitchen is the most important room in the house. It's where we meet and talk with family and friends. If we need a reason to be hanging out in the

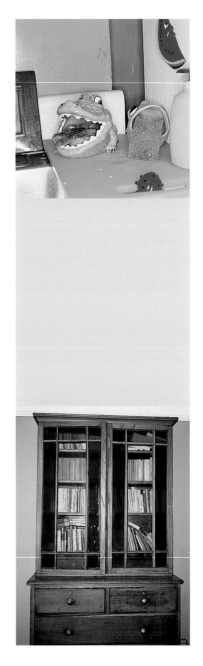

kitchen, we have one: we're helping the cook. The energy that we put into preparing our food is the energy we will be eating and sharing, so we want it to be positive. There is no substitute for positive thought, and color can aid in this process.

To encourage positive energy, you'll want to use colors that are warm and friendly. Since the kitchen is a gathering place, use bright colors, especially yellow but also orange and red. They will support interaction, conversation, congeniality, and activity. But if overeating is a problem or if members of your family are dieting, you'll want to select subtle colors such as peach, apricot, coral, and the like.

I (Tina) personally didn't want to paint my kitchen, so I've covered the walls with photographs of friends and other images that make me happy. I think a happy kitchen can help emotional eaters resist food by reminding them of the love they are really craving.

The Bedroom

This room is our sanctuary, our safe place from the world where we can let go, visualize positive realities for ourselves, make love, and of course sleep. Regardless of which of these activities is most important to you, we'll say again: do not paint your bedroom completely red! We know a woman who did this because she wanted to stimulate her lovemaking. Of course, she's an insomniac. For sexual energy, she could splash the room with red through trim or accessories, and wear a red nightgown when she's in the mood to make love, but stick with blues and greens for getting a good night's sleep.

You don't want anything too powerful in the bedroom. In general, we need to recharge our batteries here, refuel and balance our energy system. So the atmosphere should be balanced and calm. When we sleep, our deep breathing puts us in a mind state that is open to suggestion. We become more receptive than we are in our nonsleeping state and can absorb the positive frequencies of colors more easily. Again, the light blues and greens seem to be the best choice, but anything is OK as long as it's soft. Add uplifting and nurturing energy with splashes of color.

We also want to mention aroma for the bedroom. Buy a diffuser to burn real essential oils or buy aromatherapy candles that have real essential oils in them. These scents affect us just as color does. Lavender is a general overall great choice to balance and relax. Bergamot is a favorite of ours and the combination of both is great. I always have scents around; it really positively affects my system. Go to a department store or health food store and treat yourself to candles and oils. (But remember, only real essential oils are therapeutic.)

The Nursery

Here you want to be very careful. You want to encourage response but you don't want to overstimulate. Studies conducted at Harvard have shown that black-and-white patterns stimulate mental processes and increase intelligence during the first few months of life; thus the black-and-white mobiles available for newborns. By about three months, babies respond to bright colors. Birren says yellow is usually the most enticing, followed by white, pink, and red. But until the baby is eighteen months old, use these colors sparingly and stick to calming, nurturing pale pastels for the walls.

In general, blue is a very healing color for infants and children. Pale blue as the predominant color is best; its vibrations will subconsciously act on the infant, helping to communicate needs. Use splashes of pale green and pink to promote unconditional love from the very beginning. Please, don't color discriminate by gender! We all need a balance of colors that include assertiveness and nurturing. So don't deprive a boy of pink and green or a girl of blue. We need to start taking responsibility for eliminating gender-specific stereotypes. They have no place in the new world.

Children's Bedrooms

If you have a say in the matter, I'm sure you'd want to promote balance, self-confidence, and the intellect, but you may find the little person has ideas of his or her own. Just remember kids have a great innate instinct that guides them, and we must respect that and allow the many inevitable phases to play out. However, if you are allowed to contribute your two cents' worth, just give them some of the information you've learned here and let them decide. You might actually go over the different color effects together and decide which colors would enhance your mutual goals and desires.

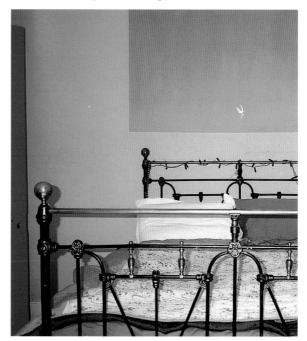

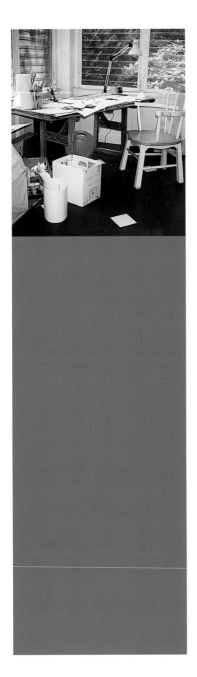

The Bathroom

This is the one place in the house where we are almost never disturbed and we can relax. Even though blue is a relaxing color, dark blue can promote depression, so be careful about that. Light colors in the coral family (a mixture of red and orange) are good. Place a plant or crystal in this room to counteract the draining of energy that happens when the water goes down the drain or is being flushed. No matter how small your bathroom may be, there is always ceiling room for a small green plant.

The Study

Whether your study is a room unto itself or a corner, you want to create a stimulating and relaxing environment. Yellow is good as a dominant color, blue is good for communication and calm, splashes of white and blue will keep work flowing and avoid its becoming stale. Flowers and plants are helpful; you need life force around you for positive stimuli. Have books around that you've enjoyed and, if you're brave enough, put up a painting or drawing of your own to remind you of your creative energy.

The Office

Color can be used in office spaces to increase productivity and focus. In work environments, warm blues can create an overly relaxed atmosphere that is not conducive to productivity and efficiency. On the other hand, certain strong, dark colors create chaos and distraction. Cool blues, greens, and turquoise are good for office spaces; they don't get in the way and they create an atmosphere of relaxed purpose.

A friend of ours who owns his own business called recently to say he found himself irritable at the office, often had angry outbursts, and his negativity was being picked up by his staff. We recommended that he paint the walls pastel yellow to promote detachment and distract from negative felings and to use green trim to help promote unconditional love as well as balance. After doing this, he found that not only was there less griping among his employees, but there was actually a cheerful feeling.

Color Prescriptions

Spiritual Room

PRIMARY COLOR: VIOLET to connect you to your higher self and your psychic potential. **SECONDARY COLOR:** WHITE for cleansing the body, mind, and spirit; GREEN for love energy. **SPLASHES OF:** DEEP BLUE for meditation; PINK for love; WHITE, YELLOW, and ORANGE.

Unconditional Love Room

PRIMARY COLOR: GREEN, any shade as long as it's not too light or too dark. **SECONDARY COLOR:** PINK for more love and giddiness, WHITE for cleansing, VIOLET to bring spiritual love. **SPLASHES OF:** WHITE to cleanse, BLUE to ease loneliness, ORANGE for sensuality, RED for sex.

Relaxation Room

PRIMARY COLOR: LIGHT BLUE or GREEN. **SECONDARY COLOR:** LIGHT BLUE or GREEN, opposite of whatever primary you pick. **SPLASHES OF:** YELLOW for inner power, WHITE to cleanse away anxiety, and VIOLET for relaxation and spirituality.

Social Room

PRIMARY COLOR: Muted ORANGE to promote sociability and wisdom. **SECONDARY COLOR:** BLUE for honest communication and/or GREEN for love energy. **SPLASHES OF:** VIOLET for detachment and spiritual connection; YELLOW to stimulate intellect.

Intellect Room

PRIMARY COLOR: YELLOW for heightened intellect. **SECONDARY COLOR:** BLUE for effective honest communication. **SPLASHES OF:** ORANGE for intuition and VIOLET for detachment.

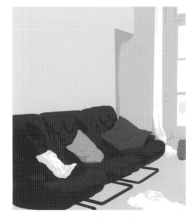

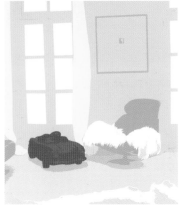

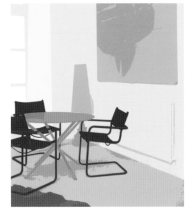

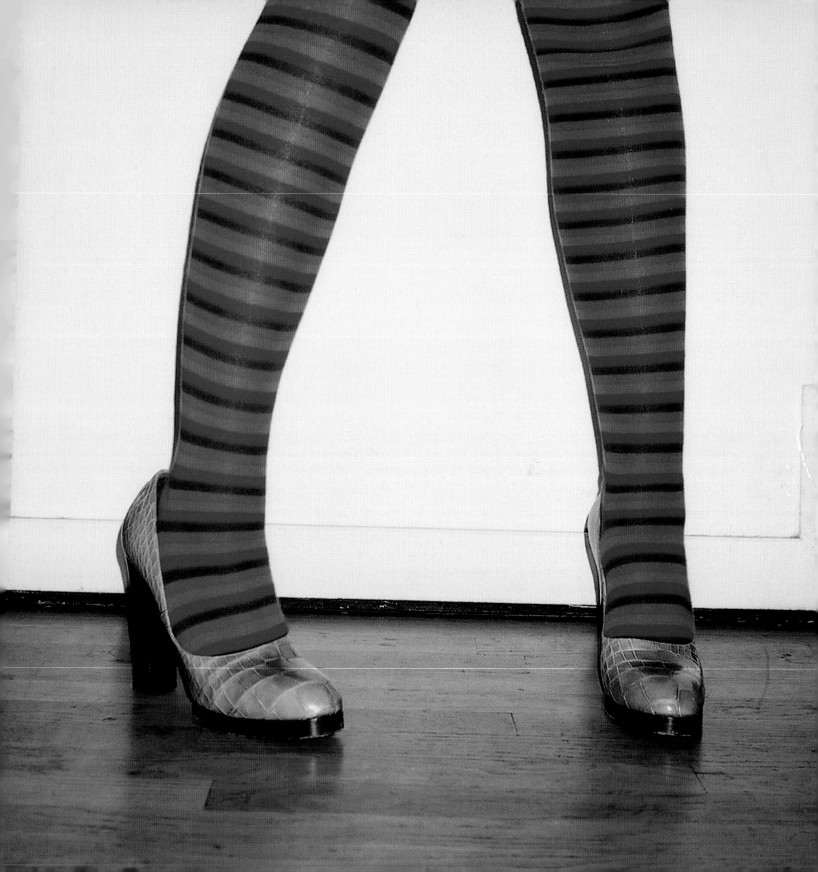

The Colors We Wear

The clothes we pull out of our closets on any given day and the accessories we choose to wear with them have a huge impact on how we feel and how others perceive us. The blue jacket reassures while the violet shirt communicates a spiritual, otherworldly side. That white top gives you an aura of purity and freshness; the red dress says you're ready to party. The color choices we make influence our mood and our ability to go through the day with confidence and a feeling of being with the flow. And whether you're getting dressed to go to work, to meet your friends, or to go out on a date, color will play a part in how people respond to you.

The color choices we make are usually instinctive. Have you ever wondered why on some days, when you reach into your closet, you're excited about wearing that blue shirt, while on other days that same blue shirt repels you? That's our orange (spleen) chakra at work connecting us to our emotions and intuition. Each of us has an innate knowledge of what color frequency we need on any given day. We are drawn to certain colors when our body needs a boost. We get that boost from color.

Be wary of the shopping pitfall. Sometimes, when our body craves color and we aren't conscious of how to feed ourselves, we go out, as one friend we know

I remember a big interview in which I found myself feeling unusually confident and articulate. I wrote it off to luck until we got home and I realized I had instinctively put yellow socks on my feet that morning. Feet are active energy conductors and colored socks can quickly and effectively aid your energy system. Because your feet and hands have so many joints they are especially good for the exchange of energy and your body can easily absorb the color frequency it needs. Yellow is also a great antidepressant.

I now make sure to take notice of even minor details in my wardrobe. They can make more of a difference than you might imagine.

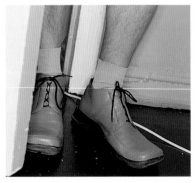

did, and buy ten yellow items that are worn for a week and then sit in the back of the closet for years. The easier and less expensive way to feed yourself the color that you just have to have is to bring the color in with a new item like socks or underwear. Then give yourself a color energy shower.

How can a color we are wearing affect us when we can't see it?

You don't have to see a color to benefit from its therapeutic value. Because color is energy, your body absorbs the energy from the colors you are wearing, including underwear, into your chakras and into your aura. Light is required for us to perceive color, but the molecular makeup of the clothing determining its color is still there, even when covered. The colors other people around you are wearing will also affect you, as will the colors in your environment. If you stare at a color and concentrate on its frequency you will affect the frequencies of your chakras. This is why people are so drawn to staring at the ocean or gazing at a blue sky or green trees. These colors really do calm us down.

What does it mean when we love a color or hate it?

Strong responses to color reflect not only our needs but also our past associations. Someone may have an affinity for a color because they identify it with a parent, or maybe it was the color used on the back porch of a childhood home or the bedroom wall or some such. Other people are put off by certain colors, again, maybe because of some childhood association. Strong color aversions that last too long can be limiting because sooner or later we need the full spectrum to run our energy system effectively.

Sometimes we have a distaste for a color because we become saturated with it. Perhaps we've been wearing nothing but black or our closet is totally beige. In such cases the best thing to do is the most obvious—stay away from the color for a while. Or you can introduce pieces in other colors and accessorize.

What colors should I wear to make a good first impression?

You want to incorporate some color into whatever you wear because you want people to sense that you are a balanced person. So regardless of the dominant color you're wearing, even if it's black or a neutral, make sure you accessorize with a bit of color. You could use blue for seriousness and confidence, gold and purple for spirituality, pink and green for love, red for high energy and assertiveness, or yellow for happiness and a studious mind. Always go with what you're drawn to but keep in mind the meanings of these color energies so that you can use them to your advantage to give off specific messages.

What about dressing for work?

If you have a meeting and want to be clear-headed and articulate, wearing blue can help you communicate effectively. Red and yellow are great for increasing confidence and assertiveness. I (Tina) often wear red to increase my courage in public. We do many personal appearances and I sometimes feel shy and insecure. If I wear a red shirt it helps me overcome these feelings and strengthens my sense of self.

Women should make a big distinction between dressing for work and for a date. You really want to be understated at work. Being colorful and unique is great but being gaudy is bad. And never wear a red power suit. It's visually overwhelming and makes you look like a fashion victim.

If you're going on a job interview, make sure you have blue for communication, red for assertiveness, and orange for creativity and sociability somewhere on your body. If you can't incorporate the colors you need into your outfit, picture the color you most need. A Color Shower (page 78) as you're arriving at the interview is extremely effective.

Dress for men is so limited. What can they do?

Dressing down has become commonplace, so men can use the colors they need with impunity. But if you're stuck in a suit, tan, black, gray, brown, or blue are your

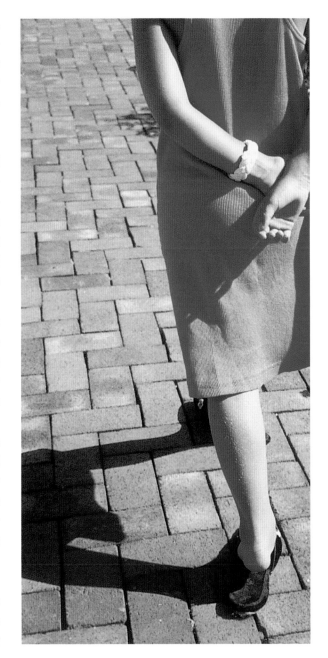

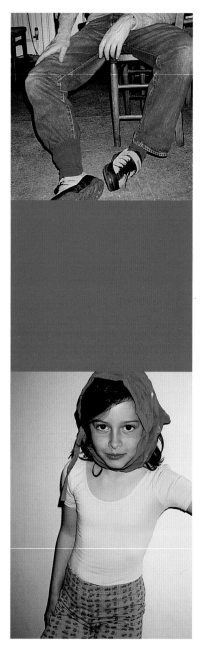

choices. Among them, blue is likely to be the best. Blue increases your ability to get through to people. Blue is about expression, and in the corporate world you are not always able to project your truth and exercise your will as you might wish. Stress, pressure, and a highly demanding job drain your throat chakra; blue can help you restore your balance. It is interesting that dark blue is so common in the business world for both men and women. Perhaps we have been unconsciously ensuring that this energy center will be fed and replenished.

Even if you are stuck with blue as a primary color, you can accent it with other colors. Selecting an appropriate color tie is important. It's no accident that politicians so often wear either red ties or ties with red patterns. Newscaster Peter Jennings's tie is always red. White, as in white shirts or white underwear, is also good for work as white implies new and new implies opportunity.

What about neutrals?

Neutrals are useful in the business world because you won't overpower people with one idea of who you are or what mood you are in. Plus, neutrals give you a blank slate; you can get creative with jewelry, scarves, belts.

Tan, a combination of brown, white, and orange, is very grounding and good for communicating a relaxed earthy feel. It promotes logic. Wearing tan will send the message that you are reliable and have your feet on the ground. Eggshells and creams, combinations of white and yellow, are also relaxing and signal an inquisitive mind. Khaki and olive, essentially greens that contain red, can stimulate the base chakra because they imply strength.

What about dressing to go out?

If you're feeling shy or inhibited, use orange to stimulate your sociability and give your spirits a lift. As one friend told us, "I feel most glamourous in classic corals and pinks, nothing too bright or flashy. Very feminine colors enhance my mood." If you're feeling ill at ease or nervous, wearing green can help balance you. If you want to reassure, wear blue. And if you want to attract attention, wear red. As another friend said, "Red is sexy, vibrant, and electrifying. Wearing it makes me feel sexy."

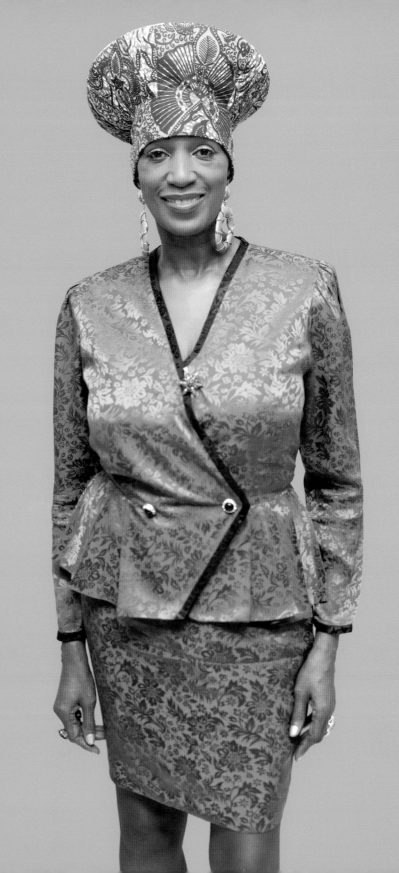

"As far as my personal style goes, I start with loads of black because I want me and my music to be lean, mean, sleek, sexy, ready for action. But black can become clichéd. You've got to take that black and splash some gorgeous, sexy colors on top like a rainbow riot. Being a proper anarchist and Prince fan, I use lots of reds and purples with my blacks. But now I've got Ms. Magic Tina telling me black represents radical change, rapid, forward thinking, and I know I seem to be continually impatient with the here and now and itching to move onto the next thought, next project, next song, just the nextnextnext NEXT. Chaos and instability seem to constantly plague me. Maybe if I didn't wear all this BLACK I could calm down and concentrate on now."

—A musician friend

I seem to wear all black in the winter and all white in the summer. Is this OK?

Black has become a staple for the modern woman. Especially in big cities, black is practically a uniform and it's really worn not so much because it makes you look slimmer, which it does, and because it's a signal of sophistication, which it is, but because it is used as a social mask. Black doesn't let anyone know how you're feeling. Black is expected. As one of our friends said, "It's pretty hard to get away with bright colors in Manhattan, where you feel like a tourist if you're wearing anything but black."

Black does promote change. And because chaos and change are always a part of our world, the black color energy supports our ability to cope with it. But because other colors have such powerful effects, remember to break out of the black uniform occasionally. And if you must wear unadorned black, remember to wear colored socks or underwear.

White is a color that seems to be reserved for the summer. To really enjoy your playtime, your downtime, you need to be free from any worldly concerns and negativity. The energy of the color white is just what you need to cleanse blocked energy and let go of negativity.

Always try to be original. Choosing colors instinctively usually leads to originality and proper color energy to keep you balanced and happy.

What if the color I need is unflattering to me?

People often ask us about this. Orange comes up a lot. But if you need orange—maybe you're feeling shy or stuck—you can wear orange underwear or orange socks. And if you can't wear a certain color, visualize it! Because thought is the most powerful vibrational remedy we have, you can simply think or visualize the color coursing through your body and you'll alter the frequency of your chakras and get the therapeutic value you need.

 In the seventies, my dad worked in a boutique in south London called Sabotage. Their carrier bags were purple with a graphic of a pile of Roadrunner-esque dynamite surrounding the logo. It was that bag, I believe, that gave him the idea to paint our hallway purple, which I remember finding a bit somber. He saw it as the color of the day and an indication to visitors that we were with it.

My dad was quite a flamboyant dresser and never afraid to wear a silk neck scarf, sometimes in hues that made my mother have to put her foot down. She would refuse to leave the house with him, insisting that a man his age should be more dignified. He was always bringing me home some snazzy outfit; the latest hot thing from America—"hot" being the operative word. "You better not wear this if you visit me at the shop" was the cautionary warning that accompanied each item. At the time I was very influenced by the style of Robin Williams in *Mork and Mindy.* Knowing this, my dad bought me a pair of rainbow-striped suspenders that I lived in. This began my conscious love of the rainbow. I was convinced that wearing them gave me magic powers, a concept my father seemed to support. He would say, "You're gonna need to put your braces on for that son," which I took to mean: For the task at hand you will need magic powers. Looking back, he was probably just concerned about my trousers staying up.

While my dad may not have been conscious of the significance of those braces, they were the catalyst to a lifelong fascination with the spectrum. At some point in the eighties, the gay and lesbian movements claimed the spectrum as their flag. This seemed to coincide with a very awkward phase of my teenage years where, due to my father's legacy of flamboyance and my love of David Bowie, I was being questioned by the other kids about my sexuality. Even though I knew I was straight, I did feel a solidarity under that flag and I loved riding in the gay-friendly cabs in London's Soho, the Freedom Cabs. Every car flew the freedom flag and under that spectrum you were guaranteed no hassle coming home from a club dressed as Ziggy Stardust.

From rainbow braces to Freedom Cabs to color therapy. I now get the metaphor of the pot of gold at the end of the rainbow. These seven colors have proven a very rewarding thread through my life. Thanks, Dad.

An Aversion to Orange

One woman who had us do a color card reading was strongly drawn to the color orange. She found this very strange because she hated orange. We talked about some of the meanings connected with the orange chakra and told her that one of the therapeutic values of orange is to increase sociability. This stopped her dead in her tracks. She admitted that she tried to avoid socializing because she felt self-conscious and sometimes intruded upon. We concluded this was the origin of her distaste.

Our prescription was to start her off by balancing herself and building her confidence and self-love by visualizing green washing through her every morning, followed by orange when she was going to be in public. We also suggested that she do the White Bubble Technique (page 79) to help her feel safe and protected.

This woman's color aversion was a powerful tool that enabled her to understand her emotional needs. Though she may not want to paint her bedroom orange or wear orange clothes, she agreed that she could easily visualize the color washing through her and perhaps buy some orange socks.

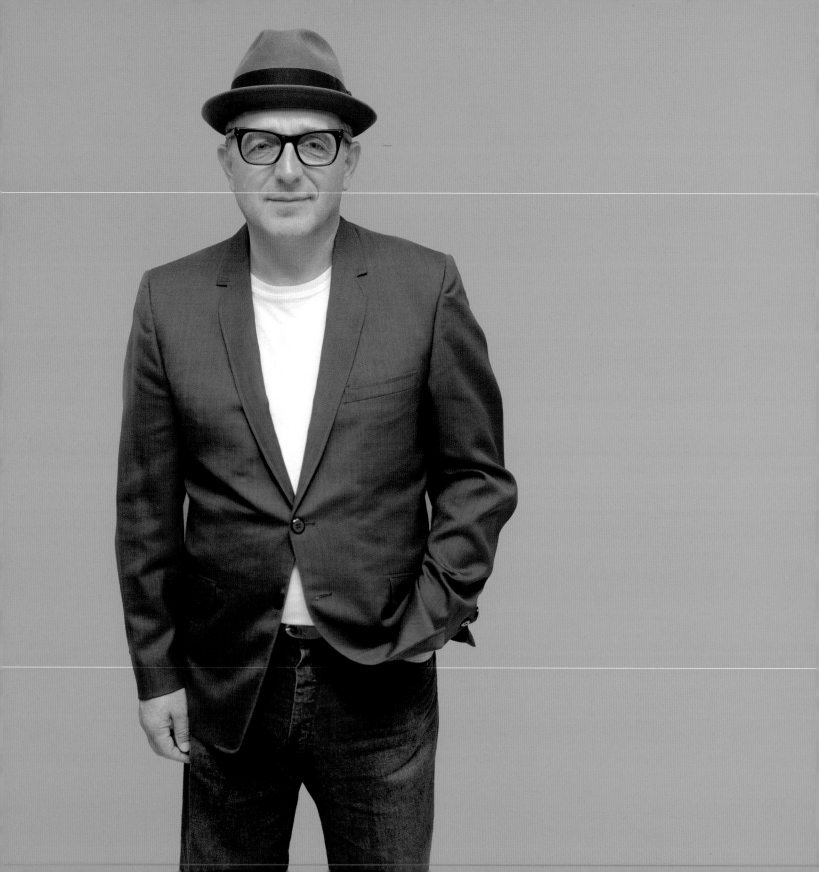

The Colors I Wear

Wearing colored undergarments and socks is by far the most crucial way to get an infusion of color therapy. I have cotton socks in all seven colors of the spectrum and I call them chakra socks. (Bringing out T&T Chakra Socks is on our to-do list.) Every morning I love figuring out what color socks to wear. I really feel as if they're crucial to my metaphysical being. I use yellow a lot for work to stimulate my intellect and green always makes me happy because I feel the strengthening of my heart chakra and I feel love. I wear purple or white socks for elevated spirituality. On days when my mind is racing and I feel generally confused, I always wear white socks. They make me feel that my energy is pure and that I can see clearly.

If I want to feel confident I wear something blue. It calms me and gives me confidence to speak from my inner being. I try to incorporate green and use it to make my words come from love. If I'm feeling like I'd really rather be hiding in a corner than doing an appearance, I put on something red. I find that a deep burgundy red can be especially comforting, maybe because whenever my dad wears his burgundy V-neck sweater I always feel good in a calm sort of way. Pink does the same for me. I was feeling edgy about a meeting and when I went to my closet, I reacted strongly to the sight of this pink shirt. It just made me feel happy. Wearing it, I felt less worried and more at ease, more connected to love energy.

I love putting on something white when I come home from work. It really makes me feel as if I'm being cleansed and protected from negativity, especially my own. White enables me to see the beauty in everything. Recently I was given white sheets, something I've never had before. Surrounded by white, I feel lighter in bed, less complicated. I feel the build-up of negative stale energy dissolving and I feel more love for myself.

To charge up my energy system, I put on my light blue silk Tibetan dress and just take some time for myself. Blue is calming and eases loneliness. (Blue should help all of you who can't be alone for more than a few hours!) I take this time to meditate, clean, or whatever it is that feels luxurious to me.

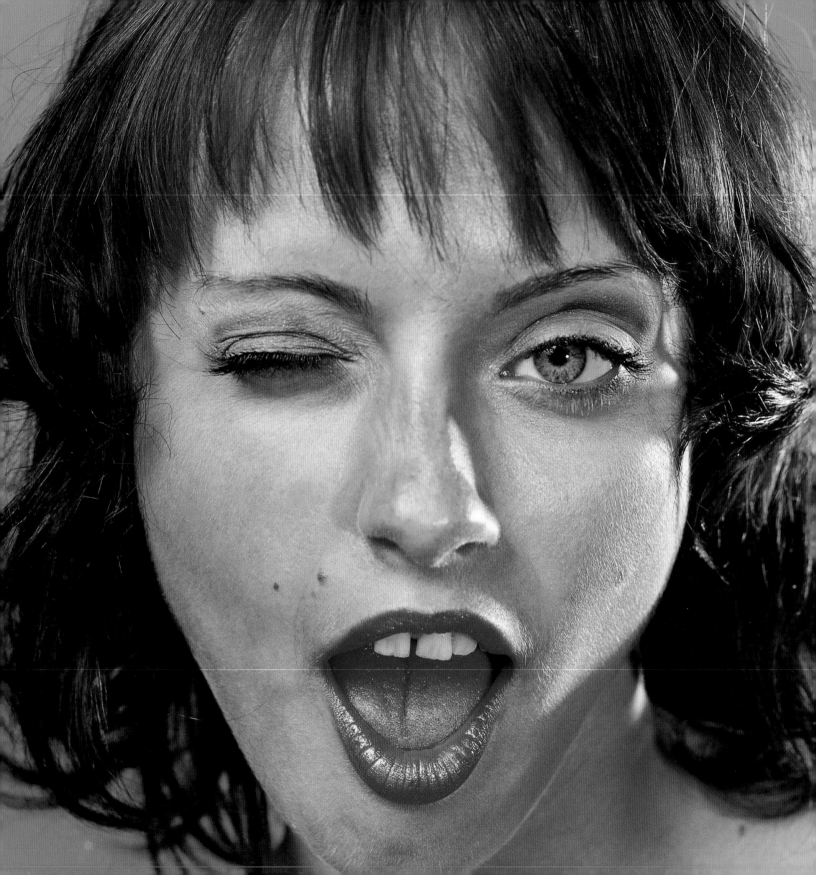

Making Up

Throughout history, color has been used on the face and body to signify everything from marital status to tribal and racial differences. The Egyptians, for example, painted their faces red to emphasize their differences from black-skinned and yellow-skinned peoples. Two thousand years later face color is a multibillion-dollar business, and women use makeup to *minimize* their differences. Thin eyebrows are in, so we take to tweezing them, but when they're out we stop. Thin lips/big lips, big eyes/small eyes—the fashions change and we follow along. Too often, we don't use makeup as a way of showing pride; we use it to hide features about ourselves we don't like.

This should change and is changing. We can assimilate or accentuate, but accentuating seems like more fun, doesn't it? Taking risks comes naturally in a life of individual expression, and makeup can be a part of it.

We have struggled personally with the tendency in this society to promote idealized, unreal beauty and we've decided to try and shift the way beauty is perceived. We want to promote individuality instead. We want to help women become self-referential—to connect with their own inner beauty and positive energy. We want to see women setting their own standards rather than try-

CONFIDENT

ing to duplicate a manufactured idea of how they should look. Our mission is to help women realize their own particular radiant beauty through personal evolution and a balanced energy system, and we have created products to support that goal.

Creating a Mood with Makeup

 Here are some ideas for achieving and/or encouraging a mood, and enhancing a particular chakra energy, with makeup. I hope this will inspire you. In addition to wearing makeup, consider aromatherapy oils instead of perfume. Not only will they be working for you as a vibrational remedy but they have a delicate fresh aroma that you may find addictive.

Confident

When I want to project assurance, either at work or for fun, I wear a deep liner in either powder or liquid. I line the bottom part of the lid. Then in the crease I use a colored powder with green to promote self-love, which leads to self-assurance, and to top it all off, I use a blue mascara. It's a fun look that can be either subtle or bold. I feel magical when I wear it. I top it off with black mascara because I want my eyes clearly defined. Then I put on an aromatherapy gloss lipstick in a soft but deep color to stimulate the solar plexus chakra. I feel relaxed, confident, and sparkling.

I finish by dabbing on the essential oil of bergamot or lavender.

Spiritual

I try to see people and situations in my life clearly. I want to be intuitive, open, and psychically connected. I try not to attach fear and/or desire to things or people. Knowing the violet color energy helps, I wear violets and purples to stimulate the third-eye chakra. My favorite way to do my eyes right now is to use a pinkish purple pigment right above my lashes. Above that I put on a light iridescent powder graduated from darker to lighter, over my eyelids extending just a bit over the crease but not as far as the brow. It looks great on light or dark skin and can be bold or subtle. I finish the look with a purple mas-

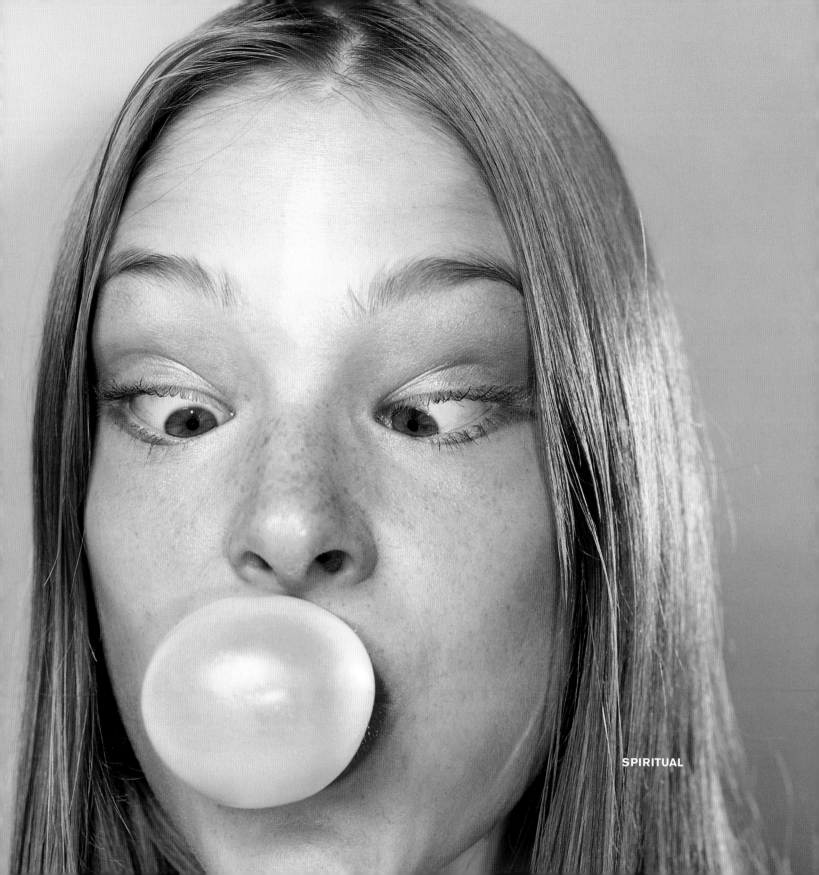

SPIRITUAL

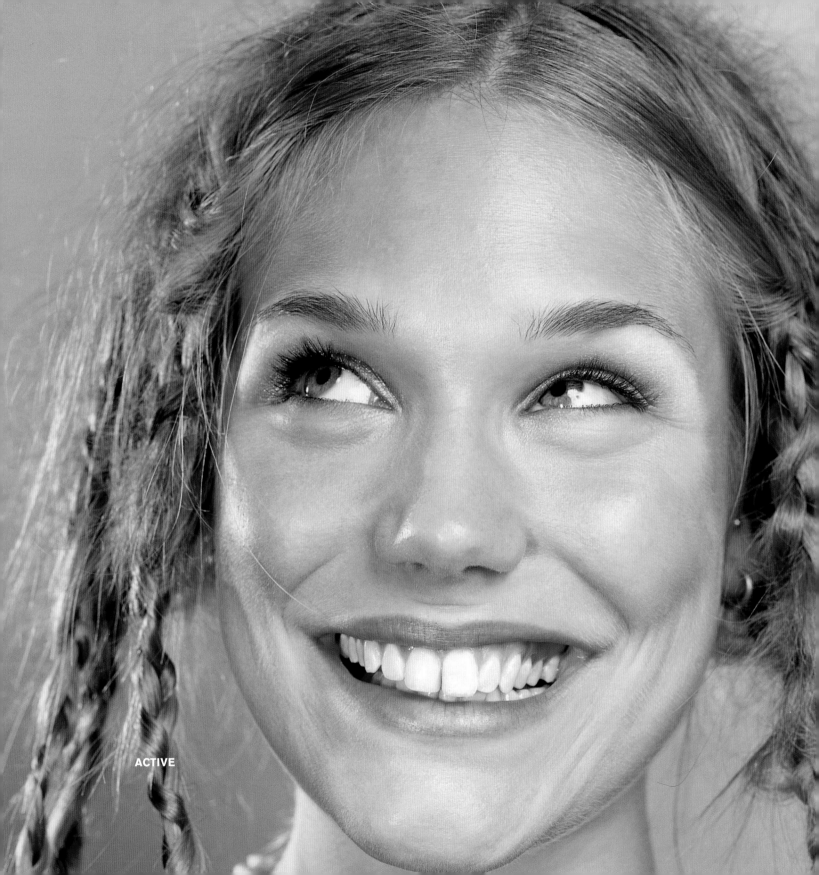

ACTIVE

cara . . . it rocks!!! I'd use a neutral lip gloss and natural cheek gel because the eyes are the star. It's all about your third-eye chakra.

To finish it off, I dab on a bit of lavender and jasmine.

Active

If you're playing a sport—tennis, golf, hiking, walking, whatever—you really want to be minimal with makeup. You could use a cream eye shadow in a light or neutral color, like pink, with clear mascara and a light brown liner to define but not overpower. You want to look naturally fresh. The cheeks should have a healthy glow. Any herbal cheek gel or blush will do, but I especially like a cherry color for the active look. The lips should have a vibrant sheer color on them. Use a lipstick with gloss over it to give an alert appearance. You want to accentuate your natural lip color. Your face and body should be smooth and shiny. You might want to try a shimmering face and body cream—a bit of iridescence is good.

For scent, add a touch of eucalyptus or neroli oil.

Relaxed

When I'm relaxed I don't really want to look like I'm wearing any makeup at all, but I've found wearing a bit can just liven and freshen up my face: soft warm neutrals, like pink or taupe on my eyelids, not allowing the color to go higher than the crease, and clear mascara to liven my eyes. A pinkish or peach cheek gel and a clear or light gloss or even just a lip balm on the lips does it for the unmadeup look.

For a fresh feeling, dab a bit of chamomile and lavender on your pressure points (under ears, on temples, and wherever you have a joint).

Intellectual

I use a warm brown eye shadow for earth tones so I can remind myself to be one with nature, grounded in reality and open to all possibilities. I don't let the color go much above the crease. I use brown mascara—I want to look serious but not harsh—and a yellowish gold cheek gel. Knowing a yellowish tone is on

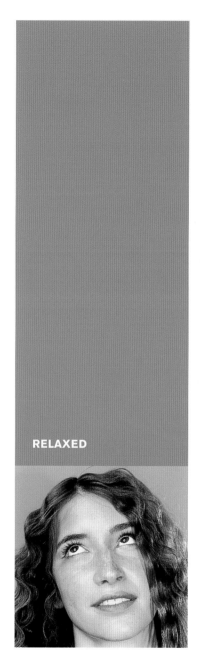

RELAXED

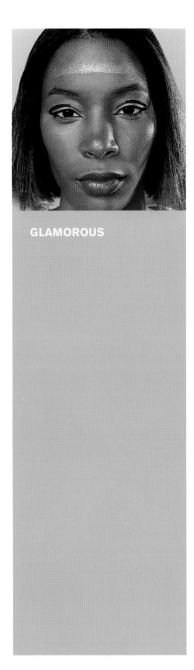

GLAMOROUS

my cheeks reminds me that my intellect, located in the solar plexus chakra, is being stimulated.

Sometimes a part of feeling smart is feeling sexy, so I use aromatherapy lipstick. You want the lipstick to be in the wine brown family. It makes me feel present and aware of my physicality and base chakra. In our lipsticks we use rosemary to stimulate your intellect, lavender to promote confidence, and bergamot to lift your spirits. These scents make me feel peaceful and ready for anything.

As a finishing touch, dab on some bergamot oil to stimulate the third chakra, your intellectual body.

Glamorous

When I want to look glamorous, I go all out. I line my eyes with a sparkle eyeliner and then layer that with an eye shadow. For extra glamour I really darken the liner area and top it off with a bold shimmer, then add another dark layer above that. (You can also get creative with darker lipstick). Eyes can be subtle or bold depending on the occasion. For a dinner maybe subtle; for a club, bold. A colored mascara (blue, purple, white, brown) can add a lot of fashion to the look. I use an iridescent powder and a gel blush and layer on a lip gloss to give a shimmer. I like to be able to see a shimmer anywhere you can see flesh. I finish it off with red lipstick for the base chakra.

Then I dab on jasmine or rose to feel sexy and think of the color red showering down into my crown chakra.

Joyous

When I'm feeling playful and up, I want splashes of color and nothing more. I use an orangy iridescent–colored powder on my eyelids (for the second chakra). I let it blend up over my crease in order to really show some feeling. Just a hint of this light vibrant color implies joyful awareness. I use cheek gel for a natural blush and a clear mascara to define but not overpower the playfulness in my eyes. I top it off with a playful buy sexy gloss on my lips. Then I dab on a bit of neroli or bergamot oil to finish.

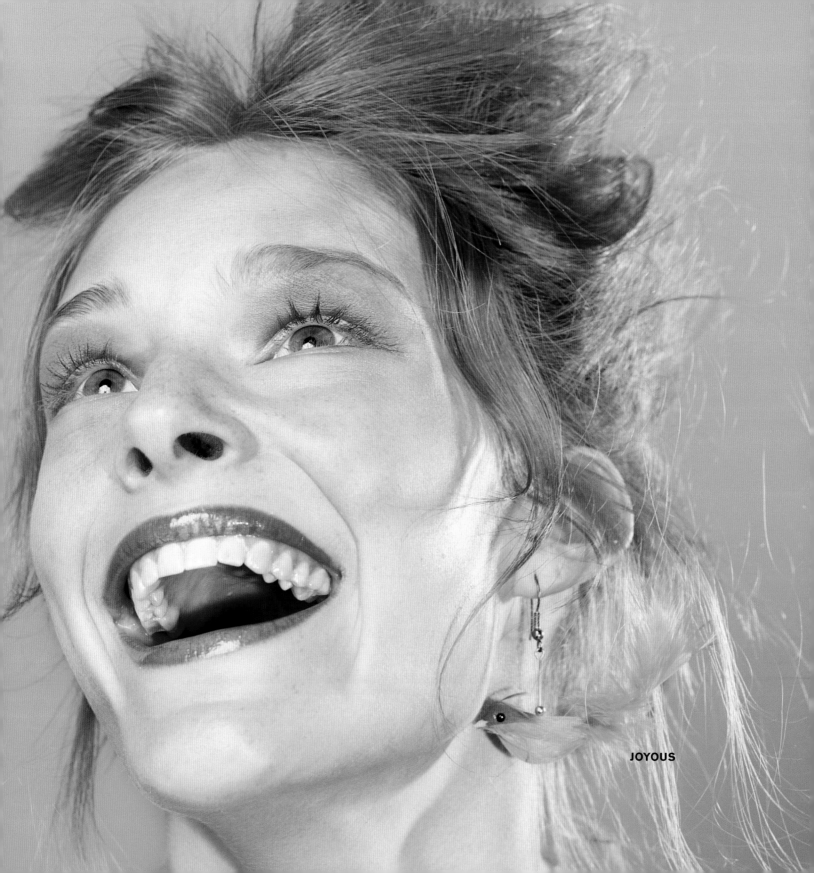

JOYOUS

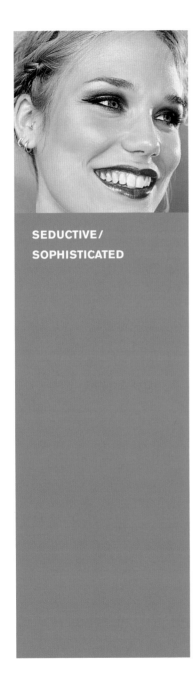

**SEDUCTIVE/
SOPHISTICATED**

Seductive/Sophisticated

I wear a green-gray eye shadow to make my eyes smoky, dreamy, and mysterious. I want to be inviting but a little inaccessible. Black mascara for extra-long lashes helps call attention to bedroom eyes. I'll wear a wine-colored cheek gel or blush, because it highlights the cheekbones naturally. A deep brown wine-colored lipstick looks good on everyone. It lets me look sexy without being tarty. Any wine, plum, or reddish lip color says seduction while at the same time connecting you to your base chakra, your most primal energy center. Any other skin that is showing I cover with an iridescent powder so my flesh is shimmering.

I finish with a dab of jasmine and rose.

A Color Card Reading About Beauty

A really funky woman sat with me. Her hair was silver and brown and styled in a very artistic way. I thought she looked very cool. She picked yellow right away with no interest in any of the other cards. I explained that our yellow center is associated with the solar plexus chakra, which is an energy center involving inner power and self-esteem. Other people easily zap this area because instinctively we always want to be at one with the tribe, so we are greatly affected by the opinions of others. Using our intuition we need to figure out where the draining of power is occurring, whether it is from a person or situation or whether it's from ourselves and our own self-criticism.

The woman looked at me and told me it was her hair. Since I thought her hair was clearly interesting and beautiful, I was thrown. I thought maybe there was a deeper truth she couldn't face. Then I realized it was the unbelievable power society has on her and on us all that was draining her energy. By not dyeing her hair and letting herself go gray, she was challenging her own idea of beauty and that of everyone around her as well. She told me that her friends said, "You can't do that, you'll look old." Her boss treated her with less power and importance, and she felt she was always being stared at. To her credit she persevered, but the effort was draining her inner power and healthy perception of self.

It's interesting how even when faced with a painful journey we still choose to take the journey. It's a credit to the spirit. She was listening to her inner wisdom, which was leading her through a growing experience. She was seeing through reality to a clarity beyond. I told her to trust her intuition and, whenever she wavered, to imagine her solar plexus area glowing with a bright yellow light, getting bigger and bigger and filling her entire body with confidence and self-empowerment.

People are never really as interested in us as we think. Everyone has their own story going on. We are all so influenced by what society hails as beauty, we've allowed ourselves to be seduced by illusion. The natural aging process is beautiful; it says you've lived. It respects the journey. Changing mass perception starts with us. So bravo silver-haired women!

We are working toward the day when women will call the cosmetics counter not to schedule a makeup session but a color card reading. Such readings can help women assess which color or colors their bodies are craving, and also identify the larger issues associated with the corresponding energy center. Our purpose is to give people insight into how they can relieve the blockages in their energy systems and lead healthier, happier lives.

Once they're armed with an understanding of color energy, women can make aesthetic choices that give them confidence and a bright inner glow. We believe our color choices all come from deep within and give us the power to heal and align ourselves. When customers ask which nail polish color is best for them, we quickly tell them that they already know. We encourage them to allow their instincts to guide them. The correct color—the right choice—is always the one you are drawn to.

DREAMING COLORS

 In 1997, when our company was in its infancy, we were just coming up with our first range of nail colors. For three mornings in a row, as I wakened, I went into that lucid ambiguous state somewhere between sleep and consciousness. An interesting place. They say if you maintain that state as long as possible, you can train yourself to have powerful visualizations that manifest into reality faster than usual.

But I wasn't doing any visualizing. I just woke up sensing this weird purplish color. I had never seen anything like it before. It was laced with brownish bronze but still appeared radiant. I told Tony about it and we thought, well, this is the universe helping us out with colors. We went to the lab and after about two hours the technician and I had the color nailed down. We called it **Past Lives** and it became a best-seller. When people comment on the color, I often tell them I dreamt it up.

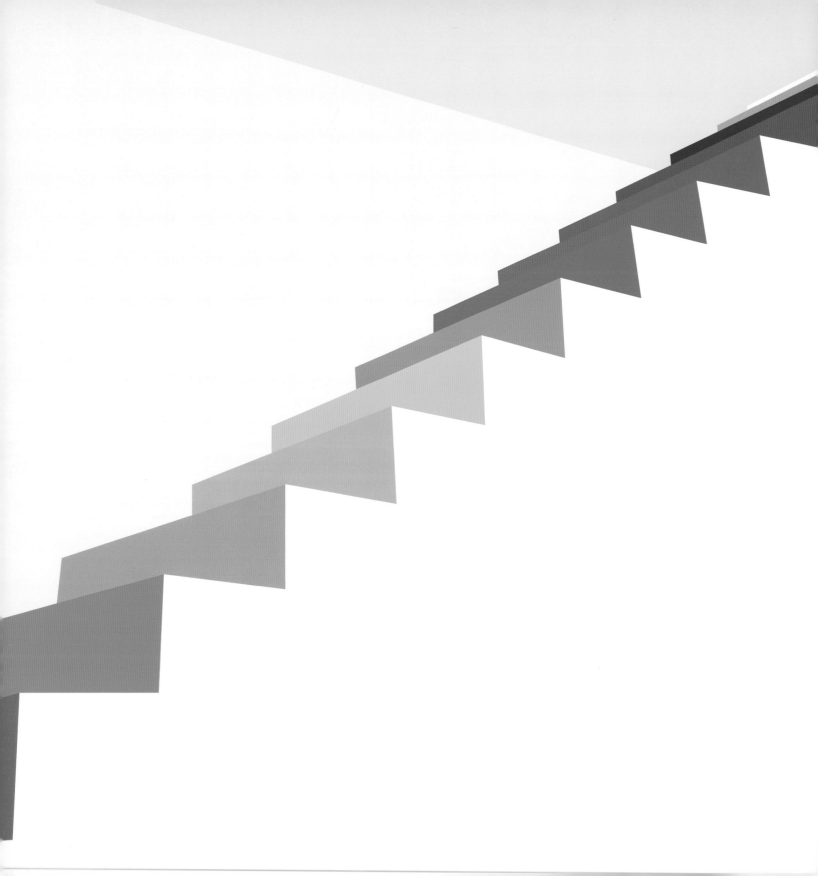

Epilogue

We are living in an accelerated time. Consciousness is expanding and our personal growth is at an all-time planetary high. This is why we hear so many people complaining about always feeling stressed out . . . it's always something . . . the challenges never seem to stop. And this is why understanding and using vibrational tools such as color are so necessary now. Our intention is to help spread this knowledge. We hope the information in this book brings you much joy and healing.

Books on Color Energy and Visualization

We have used the following books as source material for *Color Energy* and wish to express our deep appreciation to these writers for their work. We also suggest that you refer to this list for further reading.

Ageless Body, Timeless Mind by Deepak Chopra. New York: Harmony Books, 1993.

Anatomy of the Spirit by Caroline Myss. New York: Three Rivers Press, 1996.

Color by Faber Birren. Secaucus, N.J.: Citadel Press, 1963.

Color Therapy by Reuben Amber. Santa Fe, N.M.: Aurora Press, 1983.

Creative Visualization by Shakti Gawain. New York: New World Library, 1979.

Healing with Color and Light by Theo Gimbel. New York: Simon & Schuster, 1994.

Healing with the Rainbow Rays by Alimandra. San Jose, Calif.: Emerald Star Publishing, 1995.

How to Heal with Color by Ted Andrews. St. Paul, Minn.: Llewellyn Publications, 1997.

Living in the Light by Shakti Gawain. New York: Bantam Books with Nataraji Press, 1993.

The Power of Color by Faber Birren. Secaucus, N.J.: Carol Publishing Group, 1997.

The Principles of Light & Color by Edwin S. Babbitt. Secaucus, N.J.: The Citadel Press, 1967.

The Spectrum of Consciousness by Ken Wilbur. Wheaton, Ill.: Quest Books, 1993.

Spectrum of Ecstasy by Ngakpa Chogyam with Khandro Dichen. New York: Aro Books, 1997.

Wheels of Light by Rosalyn L. Bruyere. New York: Simon & Schuster, 1989.

Women's Bodies, Women's Wisdom by Christiane Northrup. New York: Bantam Books, 1994.

Acknowledgments

We'd like to thank Jennifer Gates for her vision and unwavering support. Amanda Murray for not giving up on us. Carol Southern for "getting it" and her amazing ability to manage our details. To Douglas Riccardi and David Jacobson at Memo for thinking outside the box, Nicole Botkier for her impeccable style, Monica Botkier for a great deal and great pictures, Eddie Funkhouser for his positive energy and beautiful make-up, and Yana Chupenko for unwavering support. To all our friends and family who generously gave us their time and energy, we love you. Super big thanks to Tony&Tina Vibrational Remedies and our entire team.

Thanks most of all to the highest power/the all-encompassing energy of love.

CB & AG

Photography and Illustration Credits

Color Cards with Chakra Meanings

For instructions on how to do your own color card reading, please see pages 24–27.

Red

Base chakra: The Body

This is the center that governs survival and tribal ties. When you are drawn to the red energy you need to reevaluate your relationship to your "tribe"—meaning your family and/or your community—and you may also need to overcome fear, especially fear of the future and/or death. Use the red energy to support you and increase your strength.

Blue

Throat chakra: Communication

This center will help you communicate effectively and truthfully. If you need more blue you may be deceiving yourself in some way. Use blue energy to strengthen your willpower, your true individuality, and your ability to turn dreams into realities.

Orange

Spleen chakra: The Emotions

This is the center of your body governing your emotions, relationships, and creativity. When you are drawn to this color there is usually a power struggle occurring in your life having to do with money and/or sex. Use this color energy to help manage desire and express your creativity and life force.

Violet

Third-eye chakra: The Spirit

This is the center that helps you to "see" or sense the energy around you, to detach and view life objectively. It also connects you to your psychic self. When drawn to this color, it is time for you to connect with your spirit and reflect on the people and situations in your life—to "see" things for what they are.

Yellow

Solar plexus chakra: The Intellect

This is another intuitive center, one that governs the self-esteem. If you need this color, figure out where your inner power is being drained. Use yellow to improve your ability to make decisions and to trust yourself.

White

Crown chakra: The Divine

When you are drawn to this color energy it is time for you to reconnect with a higher consciousness. White is also related to helping others. Look at your life and its larger purpose; see if you are living in accordance with your spiritual beliefs. White is very cleansing, so let it help you clear out negative or blocked energy.

Green

Heart chakra: Love

Green is about love—self-love and the unconditional love for others. If you are drawn to it, you probably need to let go of lingering hurt, anger, resentment, and grief and also to curb being judgmental. Usually forgiveness is a big part of the process. Use green to promote both self-love and trust.

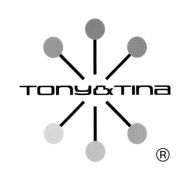